PRACTICAL HORSE
MASSAGE

Techniques for loosening
and stretching muscles

PRACTICAL HORSE MASSAGE

Techniques for loosening and stretching muscles

by Renate Ettl

THE LYONS PRESS
Guilford, CT 06437
www.lyonspress.com
The Lyons Press is an imprint of The Globe Pequot Press

I would like to thank Franz Bosch from the heart for his infallible support. He is nine-times German champion in tekking and manages a massage practice in Ulm. his years of experience and first-class knowledge was a great help, expecially in the photo sessions for this book.

Contents

Contents

I Introduction

Who wouldn't be concerned about the welfare and health of their horse? Most of us keep horses because we enjoy riding and love horses. Even the most ambitious sportsman or sportswoman will take a keen interest in all the necessary activities surrounding horses.

Unfortunately the sense of fun can be lost when a horse falls ill or has problems. Nobody wishes for an ill horse, but in reality this is what often happens. The reasons for this are numerous, starting with incorrect keeping and feeding to the breeding and the use of the horse. Added to that is inadequate training and poor handling.Only by trying to understand and respect the nature and need of the horse, can we hope to prevent illnesses and discomfort. The health of the horse is promoted when his natural needs are catered for. Another important aspect is knowledgeable training in order to have a fit and healthy athlete for a long time.

A long time before our horses were used as athletes, the Chinese and the Red Indians were giving their horses treatments that are only now becoming more widely known. Aspects of physiotherapy and herbal medicine as well as training methods are amongst these. Massage routine is a part of physiotherapy that has long been accepted in rehabilitation and used on human athletes in high performance sports.

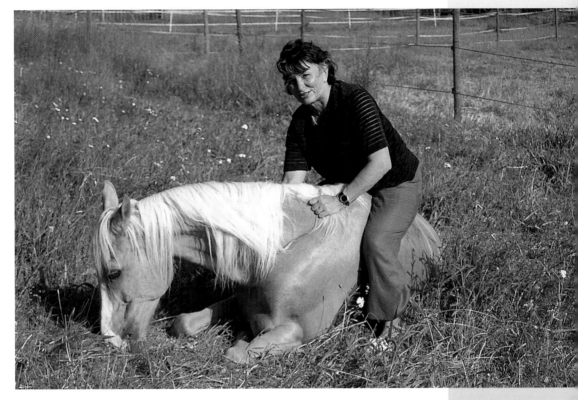

A massage treatment often deepens the relationship between human and horse.

The advantages of massage in animal medicine are now being rediscovered and valued. In the field of horses especially, massage has great influence on the well-being and performance of the animals. Another aspect of massage is the close relationship between man and horse that develops during treatment of the animal.

In learning massage techniques you learn to contribute to the health and comfort of your horse and get to know him better – a requirement to comply with his everyday needs.

Anyone who has a bit of feeling can learn to massage a horse. There is no need for detailed medical knowledge unless you want to deal with therapies for injured horses.

Nonetheless you must have a thorough knowledge of the sequence of events in the physiological functions of the body of the horse. This will help the massage techniques to become more specific and lead to better results.

II The body of the horse

A machine for movement

The horse masseur feels muscle, tendons and bone through the skin of the horse. Nevertheless that is not all. The masseur also influences the nervous and the vascular systems.

These systems are linked with all the other systems in the body, such as the respiratory, reproductive and endocrine systems. Thus the work of the masseur influences the body as a whole and not only the single areas.

The skeleton and the muscles give the horse its shape. The skeleton bears the weight of the whole body, protects the internal organs and nervous system, serves as anchoring for the muscles, doubles up as stockroom for minerals and produces red blood cells. Horses have about 200 bones (variation in breed and type) that are linked through joints. The skeleton is divided into two parts, the axial skeleton, that is the skull, vertebrae, ribs and breastbone and the appendicular skeleton, which is the limbs, including the shoulders and pelvis.

The vertebrae

The pillars that carry the bony framework are the vertebrae. They make up a fourth of the horse's bones and there are seven cervical, eighteen thoracic, six lumbar, five sacral and between fifteen and twenty-one caudal vertebrae.

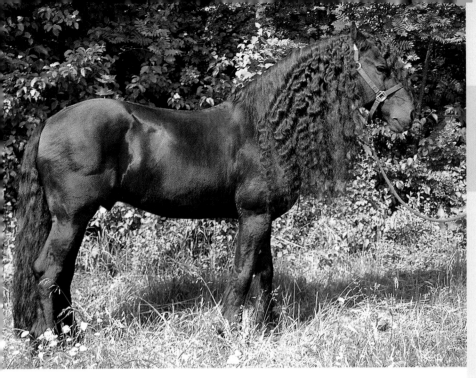

Stability of the skeleton comes from the muscles, tendons and ligaments that join the bones together.

If the skeleton is the passive apparatus for movement, the muscles are the active apparatus for movement. Like the skeleton, muscles also serve as protection for the organs and nervous system and are responsible for production of warmth (trembling when cold).

Bones and joints

There are different types of bones, their form depending on their function. They can be long, flat, short, round or irregular. The form of bone can also be changed because it is a living material. Weight, pressure and growth can all change the form of the bones. Continuous pressure can lead to breaking down of bone. This can be caused by tendons and veins that push down on the bone and create furrows and ditches. The breaking down of bone can also be caused by straining or overworking, where the bone keeps its form but loses its bulk. Pressure or overwork in the long term can also cause extra bone build-up: this is mainly known as splints. If the thin cover over the bone is damaged it can lead to all kinds of bone deformities.

The characteristic that bone can actually be broken down and built up, makes it pliable to some extent. Bone adjusts to the demands made on it by decomposing or storing minerals. This makes

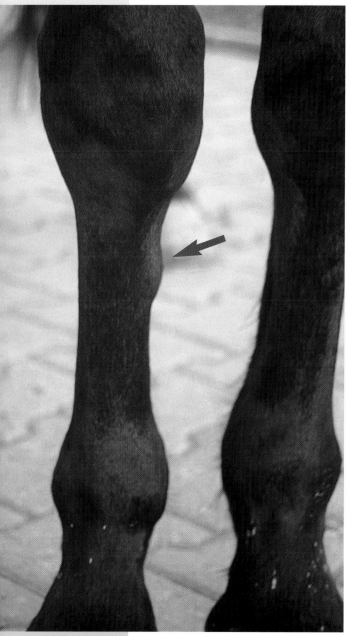

If the thin cover of the bone is damaged it can lead to malformation of bone, for example splints.

bone trainable. When no demands are made on bone, this can also lead to loss of bone substance. This influences the resilience of the bone. The same applies when too few minerals (especially calcium) are available. For these reasons not only movement and training but also feeding are important for the well-being of the horse.

In general bones are linked through joints. There are also cartilaginous joins, such as the discs between the vertebrae of the spine. Most joints are moveable and to prevent them from rubbing they are covered with an insulating shock-absorber type material.

Added to this is a tough liquid that acts as a lubricant between the bones. With increased movement this lubricant becomes warm and thinner, making it easier to spread evenly through the whole of the joint and minimise damage this way. Ten minutes at the walk is therefore the advised minimum for the horse in order to get the joint liquid warm and evenly distributed. This is the best way to guard against early joint problems. Only after this is the warm-up phase commenced.

Ligaments

The ligaments are connective tissue which attach the bones to each other via the joints.

The ligaments ensure that a tight connection prevails yet at the same time are flexible enough to allow movement in the joint. The tightness of the ligaments protects the joint from overextension.

Insufficient warming-up, overloading and spraining can cause serious damage and even cause ligaments to be torn. Injuries to ligaments need a long time to heal, mainly because they are not very vascular. Ligaments that are overextended for a long period of time can loose their strength, causing the joint to become unstable.

Unstable joints can be recognised with the naked eye in the way they vibrate, seen better when the horse goes into extended gaits such as medium trot. The vibration of the carpal or fetlock joint occurs when the leg is fully stretched. This is mostly because of a previous ligament injury that does not necessarily have to be spotted. Because of the extra demand made on ligaments that overextend, they seem to be more prone to wear and tear.

Muscles and tendons
There are three types of muscle tissue: smooth, striated and heart muscle tissue. The contraction of the smooth muscle tissue is controlled by the autonomic nervous system, meaning the action is involuntary. These muscles are used in the digestive, respiratory and circulatory systems, where muscular contraction is necessary but is not executed consciously.

Striated muscle is of significance for the masseur, as this is the muscle that moves the bones and therefore the skeleton. The muscles of the skeleton are divided into white and red muscle fibres. The difference has to do with the amount of myoglobin available in the fibres, from which blood gets its colour.

The muscle fibres, however, differ not only in colour but also in their function. Muscles that support and bear weight have a big amount of myoglobin. Skeletal muscles that are responsible for movement have little red colour and therefore have white muscle fibres.

Red muscle fibres need a lot of oxygen and have a lot of endurance. White muscle fibres need little oxygen and can quickly generate vast amounts of muscular power (sprint characteristics). Unfortunately these muscles tire easily. Horses with more white muscle fibres therefore have little staying power. They work in anaerobic conditions and the red muscle fibres function under aerobic conditions.

The proportion of red to white muscle fibres depends on the type and breed of the horse. Cold-blooded horses have more red muscle fibres and can exert a lot of power over an extended period of time. English thoroughbreds and Quarter horses have more white muscle fibres, and are the classic sprinters, but can keep up these spectacular speeds for short bursts only.

A muscle spans one or more joints in order to move them. A nervous impulse stimulates a mus-

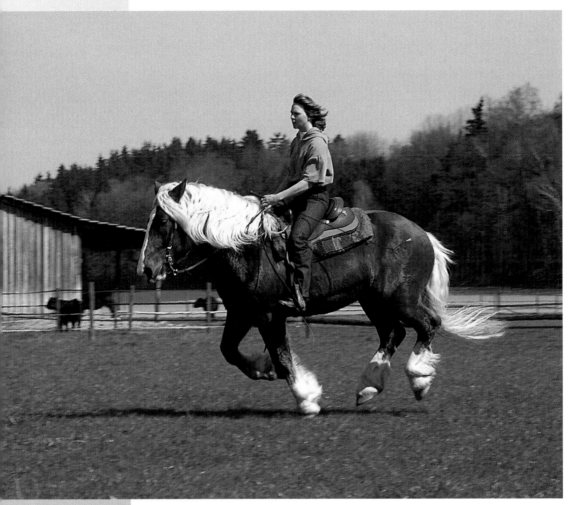

Cold-blooded horses have plenty of red muscle fibres that can exert a lot of power but have no sprinting qualities.

cle to contract, causing the joint to bend. In order to straighten the joint it needs an opposing muscle to tighten and therefore straighten the joint.

The function of this opposing muscle is necessary because muscles can contract but not lengthen by themselves.

Muscles are given names according to their functions, the stret-

Muscle mass

A horse has more than 200 skeletal muscles, that account for approximately 40% of the total body weight.

chers, flexors, tensors, abductors, adductors and rotators. The muscle doing the work is called the agonist and the opposing partner the antagonist.

Each muscle consists of a body that merges into two tendons. The tendons are attached to the bones and create the connection between muscle and bone. The proximal (closer to the middle of the body) tendon is called the origin and the distal (furthest away from the middle of the body) tendon is called the insertion.

Tendons are much less flexible than muscles but are capable of keeping enormous tension. Unfortunately they do not have a good supply of blood. The potential to train tendons is limited in comparison to that of muscles. Injuries to tendons are considerably higher if the warm-up is inadequate or excessive strain is put on them. Due to the poor blood supply, tendon injuries take much longer to heal.

In contrast to the muscles, tendons do not tire. The great athletic ability of the horse lies in the fact that it has the most tendinous musculature of all domestic animals. The muscles turn into tendons at an early stage and the legs below the hocks and carpal joints have only tendons and no muscle.

Functions of the body

All the functions of the body are connected with each other. The respiratory system for example is in very close collaboration with the cardiovascular system: the oxygen from the lungs is transported to the blood vessels.

The muscles also have a connection to the respiratory system, for muscular contraction controls breathing. Muscular contraction is of course managed by the nervous system, which also governs the digestive and hormonal systems.

Supposing that one system goes out of balance, due to injury or illness, this is bound to affect the other systems. Massage, therefore, can have an effect not only on the muscles but on all other systems as well.

Breathing

The respiratory system is a crucially important component of the whole organism. With compromised function it will reduce the athletic capability of the horse considerably. The air is breathed in through the nostrils and goes to the lungs via the trachea. In the lungs the air goes to the bronchi, where the actual exchange takes place in the alveoli.

Oxygen is imparted to the red blood cells in exchange for carbon dioxide. The carbon dioxide is then expelled when the horse breathes out.

The horse uses muscles to breathe, the main muscle being the diaphragm, the muscle that separates the chest from the abdomen. This muscle contracts when the horse breathes in, to allow the volume of the lungs to increase. The decrease of pressure in the lungs causes air to be sucked into them. Once the diaphragm relaxes, the volume of the lungs becomes smaller and the air is pressed out. Other muscles, for example the muscles between the ribs (intercostals), assist in breathing.

Breathing in deeply carries copious amounts of oxygen into the body and facilitates sufficient emission of waste (carbon dioxide). This exchange is an important function in recovery from illnesses and injuries, and to keep the body healthy.

When breathing is restricted, the exchange between oxygen and waste is hindered. This can occur

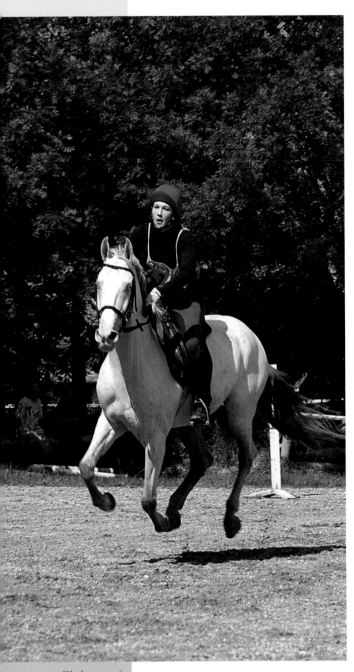

The frequency of breathing can escalate ten times with increased exercise.

> *The frequency of breathing*
>
> *The functioning of the respiratory system is also dependent on the frequency of breathing. Normal frequency of breathing for a horse is 8-16 breaths per minute. With increased exercise the frequency can escalate tenfold.*

with muscular problems: for example, when the muscles needed for breathing are constricted this will automatically interfere with the exchange of air.

Toxic waste will then stay in the horse's body, and this has a negative influence in all areas of the body. It is not only muscular problems that can cause this kind of problem but also too tight a girth, a poorly fitting saddle or even the rider's legs.

All these factors can have a direct or an indirect influence on the breathing. A massage can loosen up the muscles and thus helpto free the breathing. The breathing can also be affected by illnesses like bronchitis and coughing.

Circulation

Once the essential oxygen is in the body, the circulatory system takes over to distribute it to the furthest areas. The circulatory system has other tasks to fulfil as well, such as to distribute nutrients, antibodies (to fight off infection) and warmth to the body.

Deoxygenated blood is pumped to the lungs where oxygen exchange takes place; this oxygenated blood flows back to the heart and is distributed to the single cells through the arteries. The blood is circulated throughout the body and supplies nutrients and oxygen to the cells while at the same time taking away toxins and waste products. The veins remove the waste products by pumping blood back towards the heart, where the whole cycle repeats itself and the blood goes to the lungs again to receive oxygen and release carbon dioxide.

With the pressure of massage the circulation gets a boost that helps to speed up the transport of toxins from the cells.

The resting pulse of a horse is 28-40 beats per minute. With serious exertion the pulse can rise to a staggering 220 beats per minute. The pulse should, however, return to normal within 15 minutes: if not, this means that the horse has been overtaxed.

The lymphatic system is part of the circulation and can be activated through massage, especially using long strokes. Lymph is a clear fluid that transports antibodies (lymphocytes = white blood cells), nutrients and oxygen to the cells and waste products and carbon dioxide from the cells back into the veins.

The flow of lymph is always in the direction of the heart. Lack of movement inhibits the flow of lymph (for example with injury), leading to build-up that manifests itself in swelling of legs. When the horse has been prescribed box rest due to an injury, the lymphatic system can be greatly assisted through massage and the healing process is consequently speeded up.

Unfortunately over-stimulation of the lymphatic system can bring about an accumulation of toxins that may lead to inflammation.

Nervous system

The driving force behind the nervous system is the so-called central nervous system (CNS), which consists of the brain and the spinal cord. The peripheral nervous system includes the nerves running from the brain and the spinal cord, in other words, all nerves that have connection to the CNS.

The peripheral nervous system can be divided into the voluntary (motor and sensory) and the involuntary (autonomic) systems.

The voluntary nervous system manages the motor nerves, conscious actions and warns the body of environmental changes and sensations (sensory nerves).

The involuntary system controls vital functions such as the heartbeat, breathing and digestion. It also manages, with the help of the endocrine system, the coordination of the single systems in the body.

The autonomic nervous system is divided into the sympathetic and parasympathetic systems. These two have a great influence on each other and act antagonistically. The sympathetic system activates bodily functions and causes increase in performance. The parasympathetic system restrains and calms the body down. The sympathetic system increases the heart rate and frequency of breathing, constricts the blood vessels, slows down the digestion and stimulates perspiration. The parasympathetic system on the other hand dilates the arteries, slows the heart rate and breathing and increases secretion of saliva. It aids the recuperation and healing of the body.

Horses and their peculiarities

Skin twitching, moving around, pawing the ground are sure signs of being sensitive to cold.

Horses differ in their disposition, coat, exterior and sensibility. These factors need to be taken into consideration when massaging, in order for every animal to get the treatment it needs. The feeling when being massaged is the decisive factor in the effect and the result of the treatment.

Assessing the exterior
It is of enormous advantage to know the temperament and the weak points of the horse you want to massage. This way you will be able to locate possible injuries, illnesses and a general feeling of discomfort at an early stage and build your massage around it.

Assessing the exterior, and classification of specific peculiarities, will help the masseur to particularise the massage.

Some experience as well as theoretic knowledge is then asked for.

The whole body of the horse needs to be assessed. Does it have a short or a long back, long or short legs, does it have a wide chest or is it well proportioned? All these aspects will point to the diverse characteristics of the horse.

If the head is big and heavy, the horse might have problems with its sense of balance. A long neck normally accompanies a long back. A long neck may be a good balancing pole, but a long back is prone to inflammation. A long back is more flexible than a short back, but the general nimbleness declines when the back is too long. Sway backs (lordosis) are vulnerable to

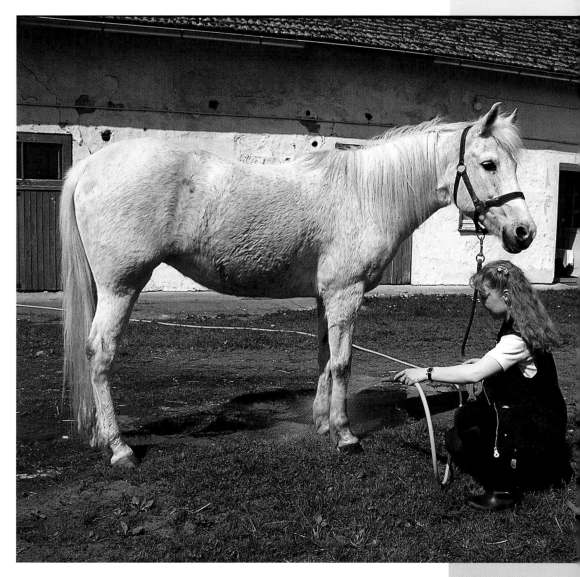

arthritic changes and kissing spines. Kyphosis (upward rounding of the back) can also be a cause of arthritis.

Each fault of the vertebrae in the neck or back area can induce tension in the muscles. Muscle tension, however, does not necessarily

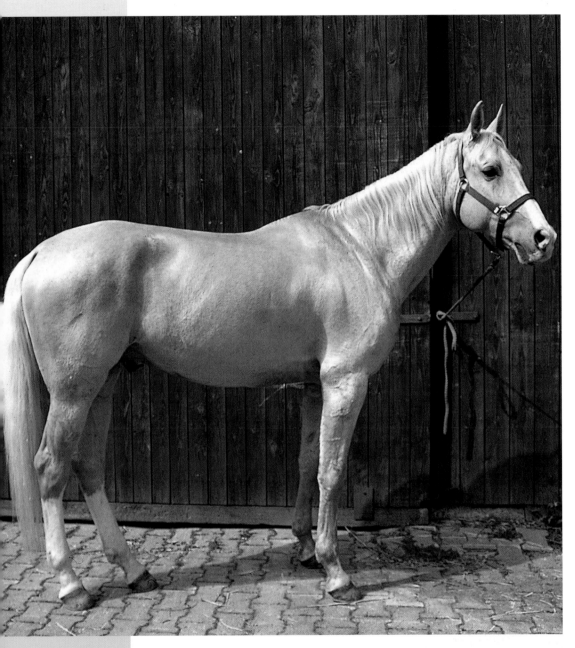

The exterior must be assessed, taking into consideration all the breed characteristics. This Akhal-Teke displays a characteristic slim figure with long legs.

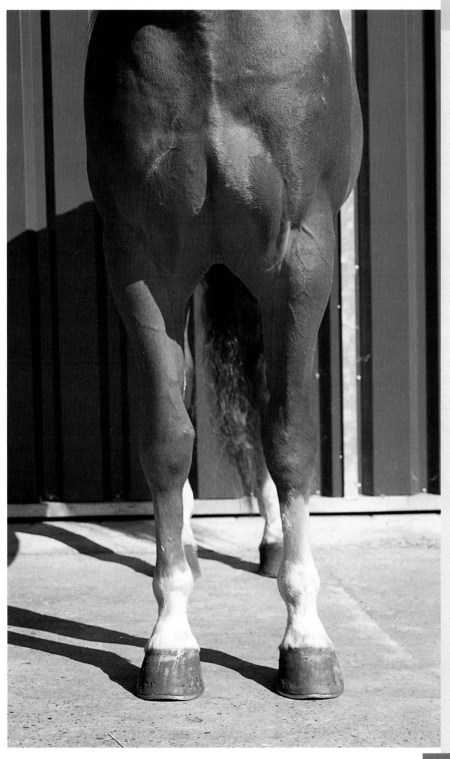

Horses with a wide chest can balance themselves better.

mean there is a problem with the vertebrae.

Horses with a wide chest often have good balance, but cannot always canter with the correct bend. A narrow chest restricts lateral movement. Insufficient depth of girth will mean small lungs and less oxygen capacity. Good sloping shoulders suggest good length of stride in the forearm. The pelvis should then have the same angle, so that the topline and the line of the belly form the outline of a trapezium.

The angle of the fetlocks and hooves must be similar to that of the shoulder. Long, sloping fetlocks may give a comfortable ride, but the tendons are under severe strain. Short and straight fetlocks put a lot of pressure on the joints.

The cannons should be short and powerful. In general, all bony parts should be short and all muscular parts should be big. This way the muscles can support the tendons, bones and ligaments and protect against early wear and injury. A horse should also have a short, well-muscled loin area, for this bony construction has no supporting structure underneath, which means it is extremely prone to injury. Many symptoms of illness can be found in the loins, for example rotations, blockages, inflammation and arthrosis.

Unfortunately there is no "perfect horse"; every breed has its characteristics, which may not always be an advantage, but use and personal taste play an enormous role. A straight croup, a short, often tight,

back, long bones with as often as not long cannon bones, are typical for the Arabian breed. The extreme

---

High achievers

Performance horses normally have big muscles and short, strong bones.

---

opposite of cold-blooded horses have stocky bodies and voluminous muscle. Even the feeling of the coat is different from breed to breed. Some ponies have undercoats with long hair on top whereas the thoroughbred types have satiny coats and hardly grow winter coats.

Muscular differences

Not only will you find differences between the breeds, but also between individuals of the same breed.

That, of course, includes the muscles, which are of interest to the masseur.

This difference is to be seen between the so-called red and white muscles. White muscles have an obviously more sinewy structure, with a tighter and more solid appearance than red muscles.

This can be appraised by palpation (touching) of the muscles. When the muscles feel tight, it does not necessarily mean that there is tension in them.

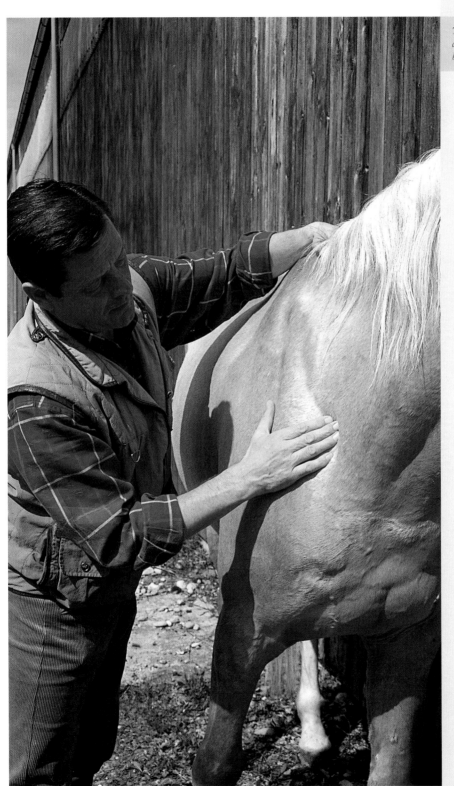

Adding to that is the muscle tone that is determined by various factors. Muscle tone is decidedly dependent on the psychological constitution of each individual horse. Various internal and external influences can have an impact on muscle tone. Anxiety, mistrust or a strange environment can put the muscles in a higher degree of tension. Factors such as tiredness, illness and competition stress can increase as well as decrease the tone of the muscles.

With the evaluation of the muscles the level of training must also be considered. Horses that are highly trained have bigger muscles and higher tones than horses that are not in training.

The mode of operation of the muscles (red or white fibres), the breed and psychological constitution must all be taken into consideration when assessing the horse. Only experience will tell you the difference between tight muscles and those under tension.

When you want to massage horses it must be apparent that you can rarely reach the deeper layer of muscles. The pressure from the hands must not cause any damage to the skin or injuries. Tension in the deeper layer of muscles will make itself visible in the superficial layers. Spasms in the muscles will continue and spill over into the neighbouring muscles. You can also influence the further regions through nervous stimulation.

It is more difficult to massage horses that have a layer of fat over

their ribs for it is harder to find the muscles that have tension through the fat. Weight in general adds to the feeling of well-being; with horses that have the correct weight you will not see the ribs, but feel them clearly with light pressure from the hand. When the ribs are obviously visible, the horse is too thin; when the ribs can only be felt under hard pressure or not at all, the horse is too fat.

Sensitivity and type

Horses in general are very sensitive animals. They notice when a fly lands on them. They do, however, differ greatly in their degree of sensibility and this should be taken into consideration when massaging a horse.

Heavy, muscular types of horses will be able to tolerate much more pressure than the fine-skinned, slim types. Cold-bloods will be less affected by hard pressure than Arabs, but off course there are always the differences amongst the types themselves.

Above all else, horses will react differently purely from their experience. Horses with bad experiences or those that have been beaten unfairly or treated without feeling will often react with indifference. These reactions can reinforce tension in the muscles, and indeed are often the cause of it.

Horses that are unused to being touched, that are treated by their owners as if they were porcelain and hardly touched, can be oversensitive and have problems in dealing with being massaged. Winning their trust is often the first step of the massage.

The pressure applied in a massage is dependent on how much the individual horse will allow. Relaxation, the goal of massage, can only be achieved through well-being. Painful reactions of tight, unbalanc-ed areas will naturally be shown in the initial stages of palpation, but during the massage the touch must become "good" and not hurt any more.

Owing to the fact that contrast-ing tensions and sensitivities are the order of the day, the intuitive feeling of the masseur will often determine the treatment.

III Getting horses fit

The equine athlete

Ever since the domestication of the horse, man has used its ability. Nowadays the horse seldom has to be pack animal, working horse or draught animal, but serves mainly as leisure activity, be it serious or otherwise.

Insufficient knowledge about the training of horses and the function of the body frequently leads to permanent damage that neither the vet nor physiotherapist nor Mother Nature can heal.

Excessive demands occur not only, as is often thought, in top-class sport, but also in the sphere of leisure activities. This is not related simply to the demands made,

Riding is training

Whenever you ride a horse, you also train it – with positive or negative results, depending on the manner and type of training.

but in the build-up of training, the ability of the rider and the commitment of the horse. A leisure rider who has little time to ride during the week and then goes on a 25-km hack at the weekend, at a high tempo, distresses the horse's body more than a competitive rider who goes through a finely tuned training programme to compete on day X.

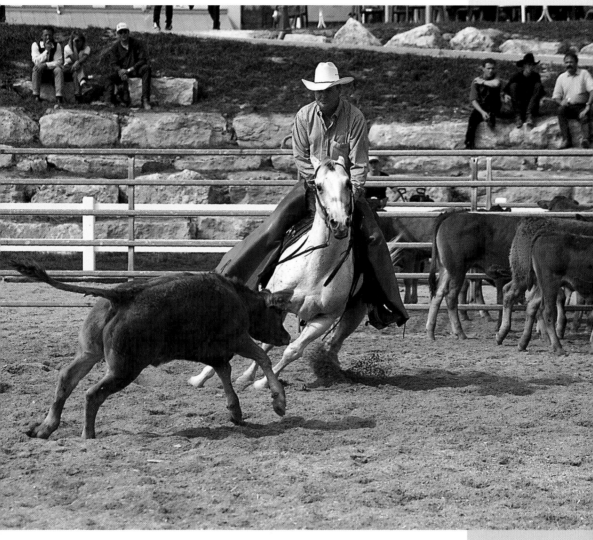

This is so even when the horse
has to compete in a race of more
than 25-kms on day X.

The horse is an athlete in every
sense, not only in the numerous
competitions and disciplines, but
equally as a leisure horse. Insufficient ability of the "only for pleasure" riders causes their horses more
often than not to be overtaxed. It is
an inexplicable phenomenon that
most leisure horses suffer due to

The ability of the horse to adapt to advanced performance is virtually optimal.

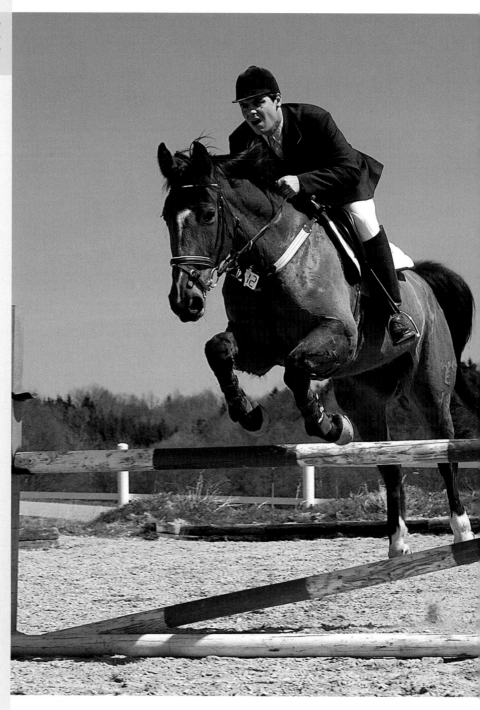

muscular or bone-related problems. The start of muscular or bony changes can usually be traced to the back or legs. The percentage of worn-out horses in top sport is considerably lower, mostly because the riders know that only a healthy horse will perform skilfully and they do everything in their power to keep the horse in superior shape.

Keeping a sport horse healthy is only possible with sound training that keeps the joints, tendons, ligaments and muscles capable of performing their tasks.

Training the sport horse

The horse is, judged by his physiological conditions, a sprinter. The amount of white muscle fibres, the muscles that contract fast, work anaerobically and therefore tire easily, is mainly what points to this.

Tendons do not tire easily, which means a horse is furthermore capable of endurance if you think about the tendinous muscle structure a horse has.

To top it all, the horse is capable of increasing its performance through outstanding oxygen intake. The exceptional aerobic capacity is achieved through the mighty pumping performance of the heart that transports high amounts of oxygenated blood to the muscles where there is an excellent release of oxygen into the cells.

Specialists of sprinting can change their fast-contracting "white" muscles to "red" muscles, but not the other way round. In other words, the threshold can reshape from aerobic to anaerobic capacity. This ability to adapt to the demands of advanced performance is virtually optimal.

However, it is not enough to think only in terms of the building-up of the muscles, as they can easily be strengthened and rapidly increase in size. The experienced trainer knows that the whole body needs to be trained. In addition the heart, circulation, tendons, ligaments and bones need to be addressed and these demand prolonged time to condition. Bearing in mind that it takes up to three years to build these up, it follows naturally that a horse should not compete in top sport before the age of six or seven years. Too much too soon will prepare the way for early wear and tear.

Setting up the training

The maturity of a horse is dependent on the breed, constitution and the way it is brought up. Amongst the breeds that mature late are most of the pony types, whereas the thoroughbred types have been selected in their breeding to mature at a much earlier age. In general it is recommended to start with the training of a horse only in its third year. Island ponies are better left until four or five years old. English thoroughbreds and similar types like the Quarter horses are often moved on from as early as two years old.

It is a fact that the growth plates are active up to the sixth or seventh year, meaning that the horse is still growing. The cartilage on the spinous processes of the back vertebrae grows until the tenth year and the horse can actually continue to grow in height until then. The weight of the saddle and rider do not always have a positive effect on this. To overtax the young horse will definitely induce permanent damage.

It is thus preferable to allow a fairly long time for the horse to get used to the weight of the rider.

A well-planned training programme over an extended period of time supports the health, prevents overtaxing and early wear in the young horse.

A proper training programme is full of variation. This is not simply to keep the horse interested, but equally to train the different structures, muscles, tendons, ligaments

---

The training programme

Planning a programme is dependent on the goal. The programme must include time frames for the method and contents of the training.

---

and bones. The plan must furthermore be dependent on the goal; it will for example do no good to do jump training if the goal is a 60-km endurance ride.

First of all you need to decide if the training is endurance or sprint directed. Long-distance riding is an endurance performance that takes place in the aerobic sphere. Racing over short distances or jumping requires an anaerobic capacity. In principle the aerobic threshold shifts with increased fitness. This signifies that the horse acquires

more stamina the better it is trained.

The horse should be trained mainly in the aerobic capacity, to prevent overtaxing the circulation, heart and lungs. This will teach it to move with even tempo and regular use of oxygen on longer distances. If you want to do a 60-km endurance ride, you do not have to train by actually riding 60-km. The steady escalation in training over shorter distances will provide the horse with enough endurance to complete a 60-km ride.

Training in the aerobic capacity gets more difficult with increased fitness for the distances must always be extended to achieve a greater degree of performance. This affects the legs and increases the danger of wear on them. This is when anaerobic training becomes part of the plan.

Maintaining performance
– increasing performance
A superior training programme will thus include aerobic and anaerobic elements. One should, however, take great care to exaggerate neither the endurance (aerobic) nor the interval (anaerobic) training, for both can be detrimental to the horse's health when carried to excess.

With interval training the resting phase between activity is extremely important. The horse must have the opportunity to recover completely (in walk) after the intense canter or climbing phase. In advanced training the horse is allowed to recover

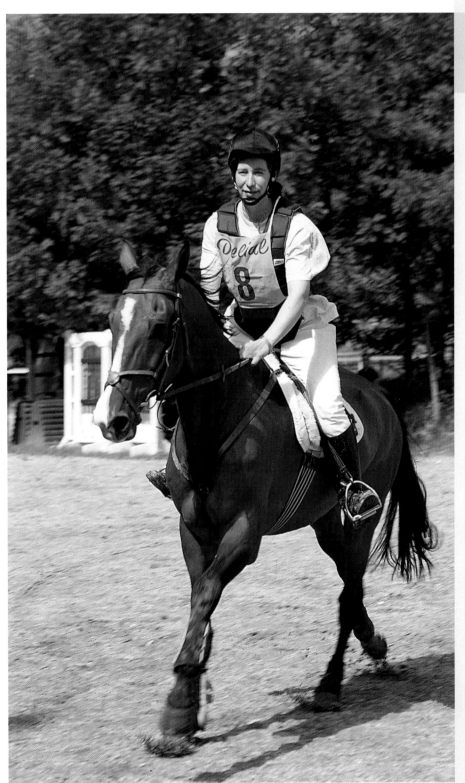

A horse that is well trained will deliver uniform performances without being overtaxed.

three-quarters of its capacity before moving on to the next phase of performance.

The duration of performance intervals is dependent on the fitness of the horse, its constitution, the tempo, the difficulty of the terrain and the number of intervals.

A training programme should have no more than two interval training days in a week. A horse requires three or four days to fully recover from strenuous training; the horse will be overtaxed if requested to do rigid training on a daily basis or even every second day. The training must also be planned over several weeks and increased gradually. A plan covering a number of weeks could for example be as follows:

1st to 2nd week: 80% walk, 20% trot increased over 30-90 minutes;

3rd to 4th week: as above, dressage work for 45 minutes twice weekly; 5th week: twice dressage work, once jumping, and ride as above including slight hill work;

6th to 10th week: twice dressage work, once jumping, once gymnastics (e.g. lungeing over cavaletti), twice hack including canter and hill work, once quiet hack in walk, put out to pasture.

The resting phases during training are as important as the performance phases. The body must be allowed adequate recuperation time

to avoid fatigue and to progress in the training

Performance and recuperation

Every phase of performance must be followed by a resting phase to avoid overexertion and to allow the horse to recuperate.

The phases of recuperation should be worked into the training programme. Here is an example of a training session across country for an already fit horse:

• 10-15 minutes of active walk (loosening up)

• five minutes of trot, three minutes' canter (warm-up) remember to change the leg, two minutes' walk (relaxation)

• 150-metre gallop, three minutes' walk on a long rein (speed training), repeat three times

• 30-metre hill, three minutes' walk (power training) repeat three times

• hill work in trot or canter, three minutes' walk (speed-power training) repeat three times

• three minutes' canter at 70%

speed, four minutes' walk (endurance training), repeat three times

• 15-20 minutes' walk to recuperate

• massage and stretching is then the perfect therapy to prevent lactic acid build-up and loosen possible muscular tension.

It takes around three months of basic training to get a proper basic fitness. A horse that needs to break its training due to injury, winter break or similar, requires less time to get fit again. The training programme must comply with the circumstances of the moment.

A fit horse must be kept fit through basic training to stay on top form. Maintaining fitness is much less taxing than building it up, and occurs mostly in the aerobic sphere.

The biggest mistake a rider can make is to fall into the extremes. After an exhausting training session or competition the horse should not be kept in the box the next day. Putting on the pressure needs a long time and taking it off needs its own time as well.

It is therefore recommended to have some light work put in the day after a tiring day. At best a relaxed hack at the walk and then the resting day in the paddock. After the day in the paddock the burden is increased at a slow pace again. This way overtaxing, wear and illness can be avoided.

The training can be kept interesting by adding various obstacles and tasks. A superb way of training is wading through water: the muscles get trained and the water protects the tendons and ligaments. The water should reach almost up to the horse's belly.

Water training has many advantages: the legs are cooled, the hooves are massaged and can absorb water, the inertia of the water demands more power from the muscles, the circulation and lungs have bigger demands made on them.

Swimming as part of the training programme must be limited, for it hollows the back of the horse, which makes it counterproductive if you end up with back problems.

Jumping fallen trees and uneven or different types of going impart ample variation to the training programme.

Training the horse is not only about reaching the goal, but also about adapting the relevant conditions. Examining the pulse and breathing after exertion is a good way to scrutinise whether an increase of training is possible or reducing the training is necessary. With major effort, the pulse can be more than 220 beats per minute (resting pulse is 28-40 beats per minute).

As a rule of thumb the heart and breathing rate should recover within 10 minutes to no more than double the resting rates. This means that after exercise a 10-minute break should be given and thereafter the pulse and breathing rate should be measured. They may not be higher than 76 heartbeats per minute and no more than 32 breaths per minute. Higher values suggest over-exertion.

Consequences of over-exertion

Frequent results of too much training and over-exertion are heat stroke, dehydration, lameness, swollen tendons and saddle and girth pressure points.

After a further 10 minutes the normal resting rates should be attained.

Massage can be incorporated in the training programme to support the performance and enhance the well-being of the horse. Massage can also aid in the recuperation period after over-exertion. This does not mean that you can take the risk of pushing the horse too hard when it will have a massage afterwards.

The benefits of massage

IV

The effect of massage

Massage not only has an effect on the physical side of the horse but also on the psychological side. These two are in close relation to each other. If the body is influenced this will automatically influence the emotions.

Even though you have, in the first place, mechanical influence (through pressure) on the body, you also have an effect on the tissue fluid and then the nervous and energy systems of the horse.

Anyone who has experienced acupuncture or acupressure will know

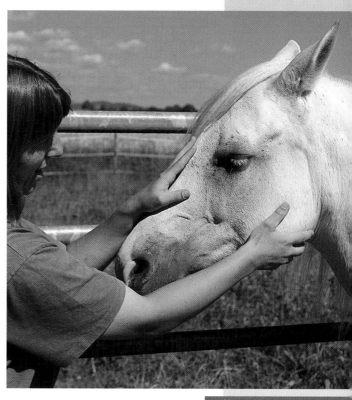

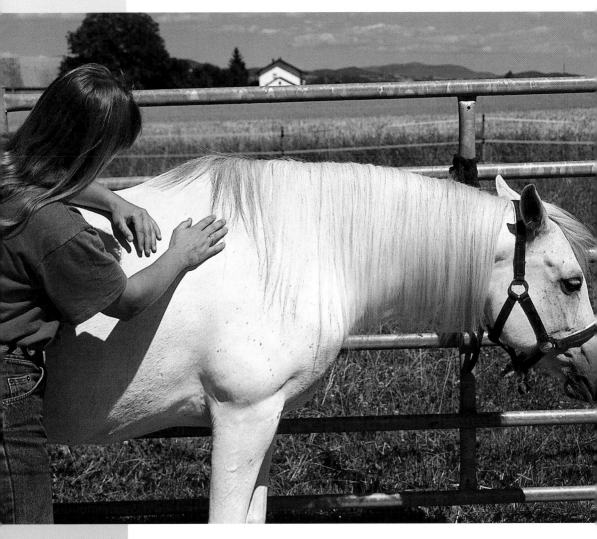

A massage not only unfolds trust, well-being and relaxation, but strengthens the understanding between man and animal.

that the acupressure points will influence the flow of energy through the body. In harmonising the flow of energy via the meridians you can actually heal illnesses. In order to have an intentional impact on the horse, it is necessary to understand the correlation and philosophy of the techniques. Reflex pathways result in other areas being influenced, which means a massage not only has an impact where you touch, but indeed all over the body. These reflexes are transported through the body via the nervous system.

Trust and well-being

The impact massage has on the emotional aspect is completely independent from the specific influence on a precise part of a muscle. This is almost a side effect that fortunately has a positive result. Once the masseur touches the horse, an intimate contact is made that generates trust and understanding.

Purely by touching the body of the horse, feeling the different regions, the owner can discover a whole new horse.

The masseur will appreciate the sensitivity of the horse to certain pressure, feel the softness of the coat and touch the composition of the bones, tendons, ligaments and muscles under the skin. This contact will open up a variety of communication possibilities, for the horse uses body language to talk to us.

This communication is not equivalent to our verbal language, but more a language of feeling and intuition. Palpation of the horse can unfold a fair amount that is not visible to the naked eye.

Horses are extremely sensitive and have an accentuated tactile sense and therefore react strongly to touch. As soon as they acknowledge the kindness of the human hand, they will build up trust rapidly.

Many horses that are in pain will try to avoid being touched, but a soft hand and patience will convince them to enjoy the treatment.

Not only does massage have a positive effect on the horse, it has the advantage that the owner gets to know his horse better and builds a deeper bond with the animal.

The harmony that follows is then from a genuine empathy on the part of both parties.

Influence on the tissues

During a massage, mechanical pressure is applied to the tissues, pushing away fluids (blood and lymph). These fluids are stimulated to move and once the pressure is taken off, fresh blood fills the spaces.

When pushing the "old" blood aside, toxins and waste are taken away, making room for fresh blood with nutrients and oxygen. The whole circulation of blood is activated and accumulation of lymph (that can cause oedema) is terminated.

The blood vessels dilate to allow a stronger flow of blood and this will promote the healing process. The brain will release endorphins (painkillers), so the massage also functions as pain relief.

Using specific techniques you can stretch tissue or press muscles together. The result is supple and soft muscles. Massage thus has an influence on the muscle tone.

Hypertonia or excessive tension can be reduced with massage.

Muscular activity can also be stimulated and hypotonia (flabby

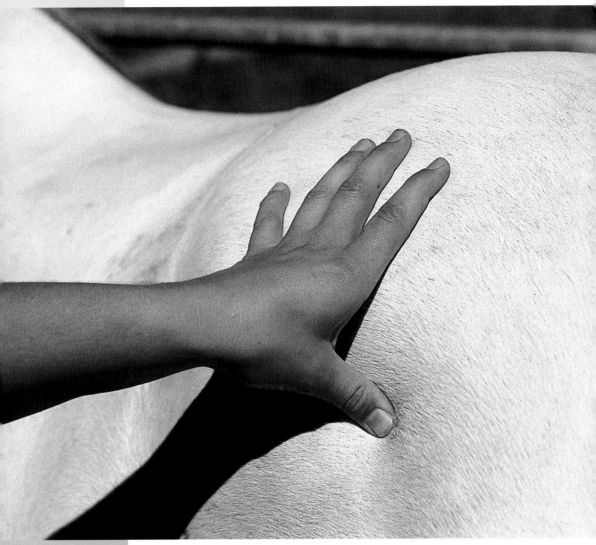

Direct pressure removes "old" blood and lymph. Once the pressure is released fresh blood returns, carrying nutrients and oxygen.

muscles) can be balanced. Every form of muscular tension, contractions and spasms can be resolved with massage. Restoring the muscles to their optimal basis tension elevates the mobility of the joint and increases the general prospect of performance.

Scar tissue that has become matted can also hamper movement. A further plus point of massage is that it can loosen the tightness of those structures and permit freedom of movement once more.

Origin of tension

Muscular tension is the perfect reason for a massage. People often complain about muscular tension themselves (mainly in the neck and shoulders) and those tensions are often relieved through massage. Unfortunately it does not take long before the same tension starts to reappear. Why is that?

No massage can guarantee total relief if the factors that start the tension manifest themselves again. This is valid for humans as well as for horses. In order to get rid of the tension in the long run, you have to find the cause and remove it. Massage is therefore only a maintenance for the horse's well-being.

Wrong posture

There are hardly any office workers who do not complain of tension in the neck and shoulders. This is mostly due to bad posture, for human beings were not made to sit all day.

The horse is also subject to postural problems where it cannot follow its natural patterns any more.

There are contrasting reasons for this. Nowadays many horses spend most of their time in stables of 9-12 square metres. This allows for restricted movement only. As flight animals from the prairie, horses are dependent on forward movement, their whole bodies are arranged for that; the hindquarters supply the momentum, the forehand catches the weight and affords support.

Movement is the only mechanism that supplies blood to all the regions. This is especially important for the legs. The hoof functions as a "pump" that drives the blood into the leg as the horse stands on it.

This special mechanism in the hoof can only function with enough movement. If the horse stands still for too long, the metabolism is sluggish and results in swelling of the legs. Besides, muscles are wrongly employed or not at all by too little movement. The muscles will either wane or tense up.

When the horse is taken out of the stable, a huge demand is suddenly made on the muscles. This is often impossible for the horse, for the warm-up phase is often neglected. The weight of the rider alone is already enough of an unnatural request. It should come as no surprise that a good deal of riding horses have back problems.

Even feed and feeding can have a negative influence on the muscles.

Chewing demands specific performance from the muscles (masseter muscle). Teeth problems can cause reduction of movement in the jawbone and tension in the chewing muscles. This tension spreads to the neighbouring regions like the neck, chest and back.

Feeding at an unnatural angle can cause tension: feed bins and hay

Feeding also has an influence on the state of the muscles. The chewing muscles are under severe strain when the horse feeds. Feeding on the ground is a more natural behaviour pattern and protects the back muscles.

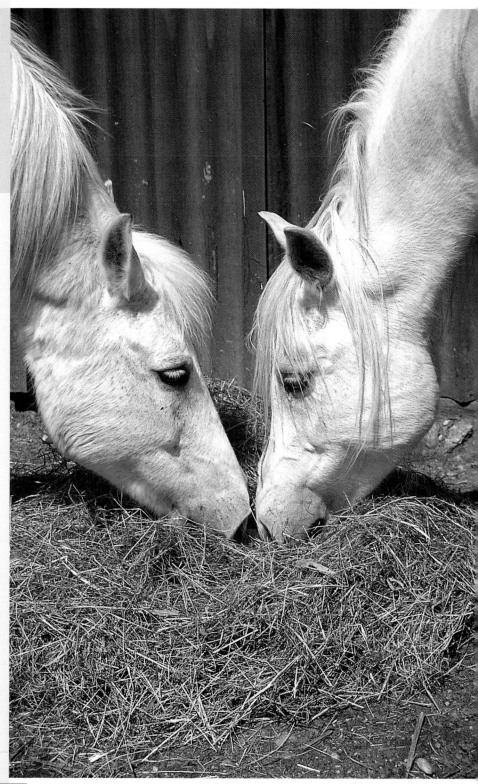

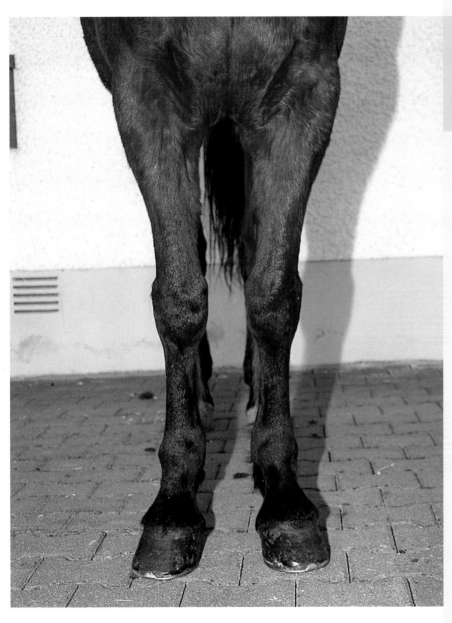

nets that are too high cause postural problems that ultimately work on the neck and back muscles. The abdominal muscles are the opposing muscles to the back muscles and cannot fulfil their task to keep the back up when it is tense due to

---

Chain reactions

Any tense muscle will transfer its job to the neighbouring muscles; they are then burdened and become tense. This way tension can extend through the whole body of the horse.

this flawed way of conveying itself. Conformation faults involving the hooves and legs have an extremely negative influence on the muscles. The muscles and tendons work much harder if the ligaments of the legs are not able to stabilise the body sufficiently. Conformation deviations furthermore cause unnatural ways of moving (e.g. paddling) that overflow into the neighbouring muscles, putting unnecessary strain on them.

Of course, muscles are also overtaxed as a result of injury. An injured leg will be protected with the weight distributed to the other three legs, that way, of course, forcing their muscles to labour more deeply. The danger is that those muscles start to tense up while the muscles of the injured leg to start to sag.

Influence of the rider
Nature did not intend us to ride on horses. This is why overtaxing them is so easy. Unfortunately this manifests itself later rather than sooner. Keeping the horse healthy is dependent on correct training, involvement of the horse and especially the influence of the rider.

Horses that are untrained or badly trained find it impossible to balance the weight of the rider. This causes severe tension in the weaker back muscles due to the pressure of the rider's weight. The result is that the chest, abdominal and leg muscles become tight and eventually movement becomes constricted, the joints are damaged and wear ensues.

This is one of the main reasons why the young horse has to be prepared through lungeing to carry the weight of the rider. After a long interval due to illness or injury, the muscles become slack and they must be retrained to carry the weight of the rider once more.

Riders play a significant part in causing muscular tension in horses; even top riders are not free of this interference.

Most riders sit to one side and therefore put greater strain on that side of the horse.

This results in uneven muscular development. The back muscles on the side that carries more weight develop much quicker. Unfortunately they also show tension much quicker. This shortened, stronger muscle is up against the longer, less developed muscle on the other side and therefore the horse will find it easier to bend to the stronger side.

Ultimately this influences the length of the steps and general balance of the horse. This imbalance delivers us back to tension and pressure in the different regions.

Worst sinners of all are the bad riders who cannot compensate for their bad seat by balancing in the movement. They fall into the horse's back muscles with every step (especially in trot and canter), and naturally this pain will cause the horse to lower its back and tense up its muscles.

Clinging legs from the rider will furthermore make the horse tense up its stomach muscles.

A hard hand and tight rein will create tension in the neck, chest and back muscles. Advanced riders

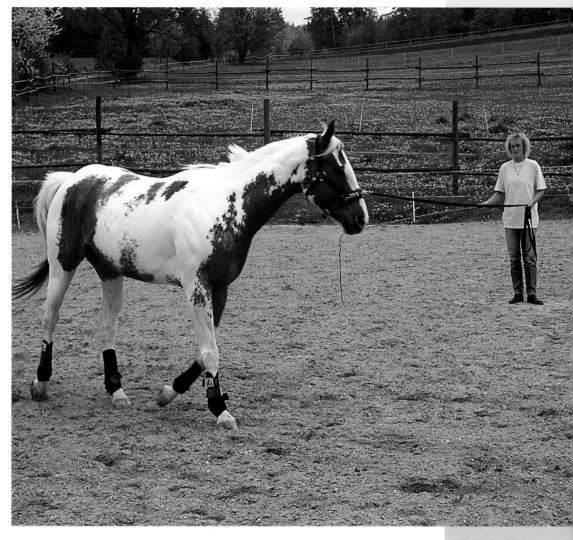

The muscles of the young horse must be prepared to carry the weight of the rider through careful lungeing.

can summon up tension if they do not allow the horse the chance to stretch during training.

Every time a muscle is overtaxed it will tense up even more because it does not have the chance to recover. Shaping the muscle is only possible when the effort is alternated with relaxation. Long-lasting contraction will lead to tightening up of the muscles.

Saddles that fit badly can also contribute to tension in the muscles, not to mention ill-fitting bridles and equipment. It is the rider's responsibility to ensure the equipment used on the horse fits properly and serves the purpose.

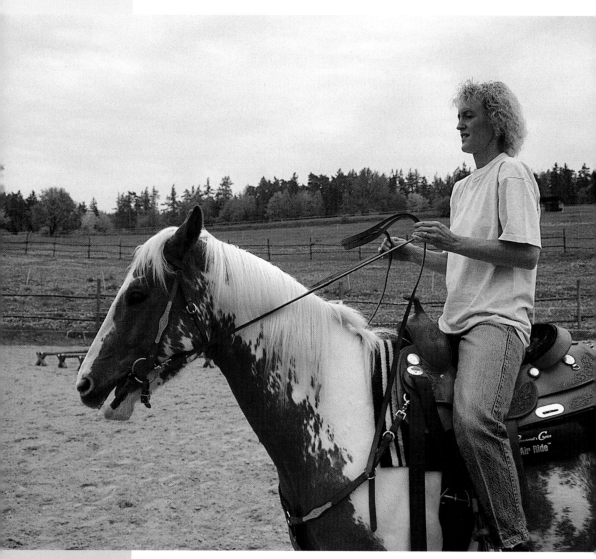

The rider plays a significant part in the tension of the horse's muscles. An unbalanced seat and hard hand influence tension in the horse's neck and back.

It is the rider's duty to train himself to the highest possible niveau in order to protect the horse from unnecessary injury that can be caused by the imbalance of the rider. Massage treatments can relieve pain and help the well-being of the horse, but unfortunately it is not possible to compensate for the faults made by the rider or poorly fitting tack. Massage is simply a supporting therapy.

Practical application

While every horse feels different, it is also important to adapt the massage techniques to the horse. Not only do the sensitivity, character and type of horse dictate the massage, but the state of health and the goal of the massage play important roles as well.

By using the different massage techniques you can achieve various effects that support the well-being, enhance the performance and overcome injury rapidly.

The result is not the only reason for choosing a specific massage technique; you have to consider the situation in general to obtain an optimal result. The massage techniques can in general be categorised and be used to your advantage if you do not yet have enough experience in the massage of horses.

You must always talk to the vet before giving a horse a therapeutic massage. Illness or injury can seldom be healed through massage alone, but massage can certainly aid and support the process.

As a rule, the relaxing, preventive massage is used for the pleasure it gives horses and to raise their feelings of well-being. Once you have more experience with the different strokes and techniques you can apply them with more effect.

Relaxation and suppling
Horses are flight animals by nature and because of this, situations of stress can easily cause tensions in their muscles.

The pressure of performance under saddle and bad posture (feeding too high, boredom and trouble with other horses in the paddock) are stress factors that can lead to aggression and feeling indisposed. If these conditions cannot be improved upon, at least the stress can be relieved with a relaxing massage.

The relaxing massage can be put to good use in short stressful situations such as travelling in a box.

This relaxing massage is a technique that can be used any time for it is a component of further techniques. It also serves to build the contact and relationship between horse and human.

Long, flowing strokes (effleurage) are used for the relaxation massage. The pressure must not be too strong, so that it will not show any reaction of pain or irritation. The whole massage takes 15-20 minutes. These long, slow strokes act in a relaxing way, whereas fast strokes will wake and stimulate the horse.

Prevention and increase of performance
The relaxation massage can precede any type of massage. A further massage that protects the horse from strong muscle tension (that reveals tightness at an early stage) and keeps it in a fit state where performance is achievable, is the maintenance massage.

Using this preventive massage can reveal the smallest pressure and stress points before they be-

The basic stroke used in the relaxation massage is a long, flowing move made with the hands and fingers.

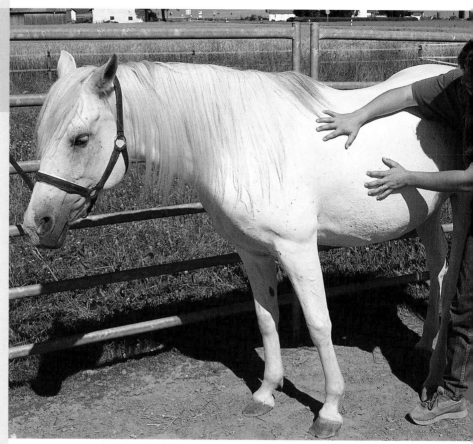

come serious. It is especially important for sport horses that preventive measures are taken in order to avoid the tension and pain that goes with it. Muscular illness or injury puts the sport horse out of action; training is interrupted and has to be rebuilt after long periods of rest. Such interruptions can be avoided if the tensions are treated promptly.

The maintenance massage incorporates kneading, compression, friction and vibration, alternated

Real relaxation

The relaxation massage is done using long and relaxing strokes.

with the long stroking moves. Each muscle undergoes an examination and the treatment follows this assessment.

The preventive massage is the basic treatment for all horses. None of these techniques is set in stone and they can be adapted to comply with the needs of each individual horse.

The purpose of the massage determines in the first instance how you massage and what techniques will be used.

This means that even the maintenance massage is no specific technique, but varies according to need.

An exhausted, tired horse will be massaged with faster strokes and kneading to get the energy flowing while a nervous horse will profit more from the soft, slow strokes of a relaxing massage.

Illness and injury

The specific massage used to treat illness and injury has a special role. Before any treatment, however, the vet must be consulted to diagnose the illness or injury.

The therapy plan can be developed once the diagnosis has been made. This can be done with the help of the vet, a physiotherapist

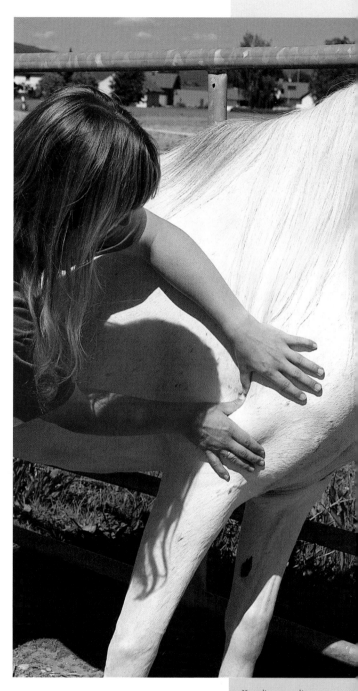

Kneading can relieve and prevent tension and is often used in maintenance massage.

*Each individual
muscle is examined
and treated with
kneading and
compression.*

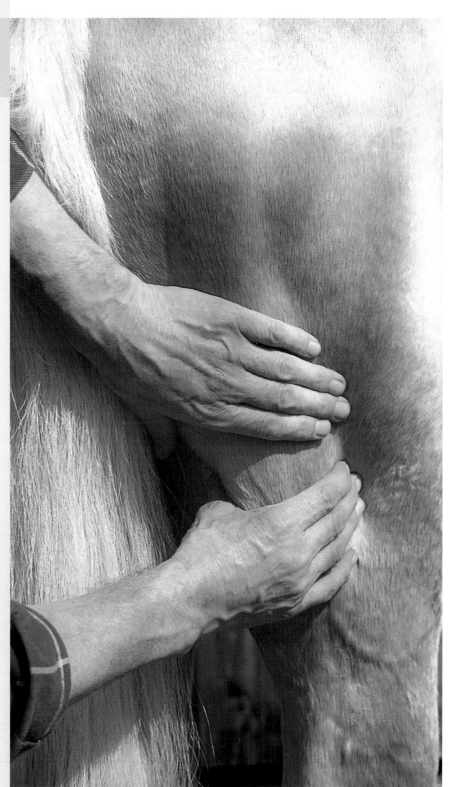

and massage therapist and the final plan of action must always be discussed with the vet.

As a rule, massage can assist in promoting recovery from injury, for it is about increasing the flow of blood and removal of waste products. Massage can of course cause damage in certain cases, for example massage is contra-indicated in acute injuries where warmth, swelling and inflammation are present. These injured areas must then be excluded from the treatment. (For contra-indications, see p. 71.)

Apart from acute injuries, massage can be successfully applied to smoothe scar tissue. Cross-friction, circular movement, kneading and rolling of the skin is used to promote this. Scar tissue is usually the result of injuries, which means this treatment will support the rehabilitation.

When swollen legs are a problem, it is mostly the lymphatic system that is overstretched. The lymphatic system is no longer capable of transporting all the waste, and the result is swollen legs. Swollen legs are generally a sign of the body being overtaxed, but standing still too long (due to an injury or illness) can also contribute to this condition. The use of the muscles is necessary for the flow of lymph, which in effect means that no muscular movement will have a negative influence on the lymphatic flow.

Once the horse is moving, swollen legs tend to disappear. Massage is a superb way to get the lymph flowing again. Stroking the legs in an upward direction (against the

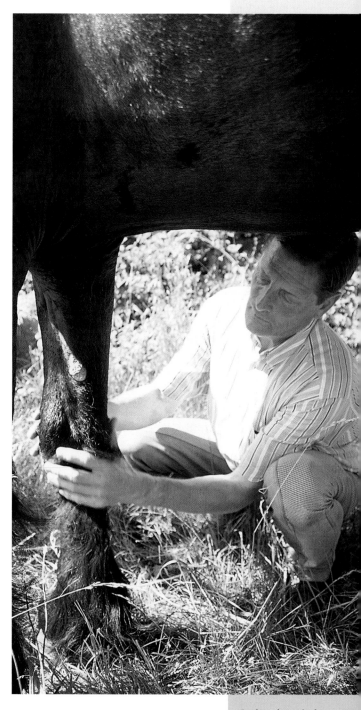

Stroking the inside of the leg in the direction of the heart will get the lymph flowing again.

hair) helps the flow of lymph, for it must travel in the direction of the heart. This is a way of preventing or removing lymphatic build-up.

After training and competition
Most riders accept proper warming-up of the horse's muscles as a matter of course in order to prepare the horse for the burden that follows. Unfortunately too little time and thought is given to the cooling-down phase after the effort.

Too many horses are simply put back into the stable after a competition or training. They are seldom allowed to relax and cool down after the exertion. The cooling of the body and getting the pulse rate back to normal can take up to 20 minutes.

Putting the horse in the stable too soon will increase the collection of lactic acid in the body and will result in the hardening of the muscles.

The cooling-down period is therefore as important as the warm-up phase. The muscles must be allowed to relax and return to their normal state.

A massage to relax and revive can assist the muscles to loosen and drain away waste through stimulation of the circulation. This will impel the lymph to move and the danger of swollen legs will be dramatically reduced.

Massage can reduce the time needed to regenerate, helping the horse to continue its high level of performance more rapidly.

Do not, however, be tempted to shorten the cooling-down phase

---

Stay moving

Insufficient time to cool down will cause lactic acid to build up in the muscles.

---

because you are massaging the horse afterwards.

The lowering of the pulse and breathing is important before having a massage, for massage is no substitute for the cooling-down, but a complement.

Massage comprises in the first place the removal of waste products from the tissues, more specifically the lymph and then mainly in the back and leg area. In the lymphatic capillaries, you will find lymph nodes where toxins get filtered out of the system. There is a bigger concentration of these glands on the inside of the limbs. By using soft stroking moves in these areas as well as soft vibration and shaking, you can promote the flow of lymph in the direction of the heart.

You commence the aftercare massage in the area of the withers and back. Stroking along the vertebrae promotes circulation and kneading will loosen the muscles.

Next you move on to the chest area. Run your fingers along the ribs in the direction of the limbs. Do some cupping (hand held slightly cupped with fingers together) to draw the lactic acid out of the deeper layers. With hand stroking you then work from the shoulder around to the front of the chest, employing extensive kneading and shaking as well.

To drain the tissue of excess liquid, stroke the legs from the bottom up and give preference to the insides of the legs. This leads on to the stroking of the neck and compression and kneading in the area of the mane. When the horse lowers its head you are working with the correct intensity. On the head you stroke the jaw and underside of the neck. Finally you apply long, slow strokes over the whole body of the horse.

V

Massage techniques

Tracking down tension

The main purpose of massage is the prevention and rectification of tension and knots in the muscles. Due to the fact that the muscles transmit their tension to their neighbours, it is always better to massage the whole body. There are of course times when localised treatments can be done, especially the areas that are prone to tension due to breed or discipline (see Problem Areas, p.92).

Each individual horse can develop its own problems arising from the conformation, discipline, training and influence from the rider. Complete assessment of the whole horse will point to the specific areas that

might call for particular attention to prevent tension and scar tissue from setting in.

Effleurage exploration
The exploration of the body assists both in pinpointing tension and gaining the trust of the horse. Once you have a clear picture of the horse's body you can treat it more meticulously, which is crucial in averting any contra-indications in the maintenance massage.

Exploration with effleurage is the stroking of the horse's body, investigating the skin, muscle tone and temperature. By applying light

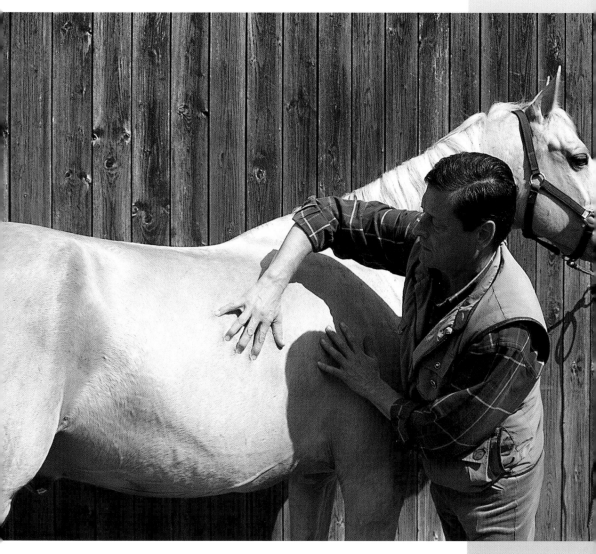

Stroking with the hands and fingers make you aware of the tone of the muscles, temperature and condition of the horse.

pressure you can sense spasms and knots and remove them.

Stroking with the hands is at the same time draining the tissues and can easily be used in the transition to the maintenance or relaxation massage.

Caress with care

The foundation of massage is stroking with the hands and fingers, and using them to make the transition from one area to another.

Effleurage is the ideal way to commence a massage and also the best way to end it. After every massage technique and change-over to another area of the body, effleurage can be employed. Effleurage is the backbone of every massage.

In assessing the body, you start by stroking at the head and continue over the neck, back, barrel and legs of the horse.

Wherever muscle transforms into tendons, the compression must be relieved, for most pressure points are found there, being revealed as gritty, round or even stringy tissue.

Tension in the shoulder can also be found behind the shoulder blade. Owing to the fact that the shoulder (and indeed the complete forelimb) is not attached to the body with a joint but only through muscle and tendons, the shoulder blade is easily lifted when the muscles are relaxed.

When the muscles surrounding the shoulder blade are relaxed, it is possible to slip the whole of your flat hand into the area behind the shoulder blade. However, when tension is present you can at the very most insert only one or two fingers.

An additional area to test for tension is the tail. If the dock of the tail can comfortably be bent up or sideways, it is a sign that there is no extreme tension in the area of the back. If it is difficult to lift the dock of the tail, the possibility of tension in the back is greater.

The dock must never be lifted by force, but rather after a complete

relaxing massage. If in doubt, it is always better to call the vet, for an unusually stiff tail can point to extreme injury.

Massage movements

In order to compile a treatment plan for your horse, you must have sufficient knowledge of the different movements, when to use them and what their results are. Every movement can have a different effect by changing the pressure or speed with which they are executed.

The outcome is also affected by the feeling from the masseur, particularly when the movements must still be learnt. In many instances, the same objective can be achieved with varying techniques. This is why it is important to know why a technique is used and what the results are likely to be.

Depending on your personal preference, strength and skill you can, for example, employ pressure with a thumb, two fingers or an elbow. A certain amount of experience will be required to find the right amount of pressure and speed that will accompany the optimum results.

Hand and finger stroking
No strength is required to utilise this technique. It is a light touch, that seldom entails more than 1kg of pressure.

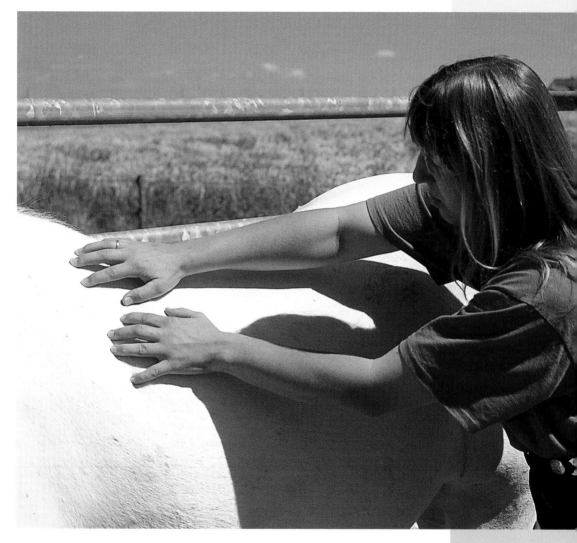

Finger stroking is pulling the fingertips towards your own body in the direction of the growth of the hair.

If a deep massage is required the pressure can be increased to 5kg or more. To test the physical force needed, you can use a kitchen or bathroom scale, for you can easily be deceived by what you perceive as pressure and the actual load.

Finger stroking is when you put your spread fingertip on the horse's body and pull them in the direction of the hair (and towards your body!) over the horse. The whole hand, including the palm, has contact with the horse's body when hand

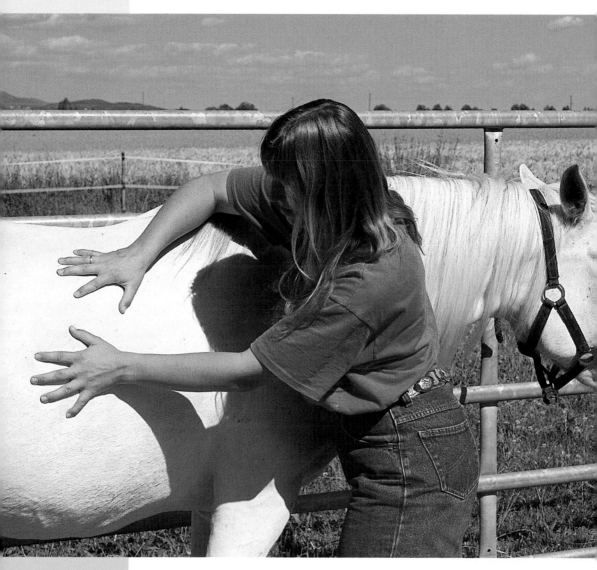

Hand stroking is pushing the hands away from your body, staying in the direction of the growth of the hair.

stroking is used. Unlike finger stroking, you push the hands away from your body when using hand stroking. These techniques can be used over the whole body, easing up over bony structures and applying more pressure on the muscular areas.

The stroking can be repeated 10-20 times over every part of the body, using both hands.

Stroking has a pain relieving, relaxing and calming effect and is used as the main technique in relaxation massage. Fast strokes have a stimulating effect and wake up the body, which means the relaxing strokes must be slow and expressive. Hand stroking influences the lymphatic flow and can be utilised to drain the tissue and combat swelling of the legs.

Hand and finger stroking initiate every massage, serve as a bridging technique when you move to another type of movement and conclude each massage.

Effleurage additionally serves to uncover tension, spasms and knots and thus acts as both a diagnostic and therapeutic technique.

Every horse owner has applied – even without knowing it – stroking techniques. Grooming the horse is nothing but stroking the body with a brush, achieving the same results as with the hand. The difference is

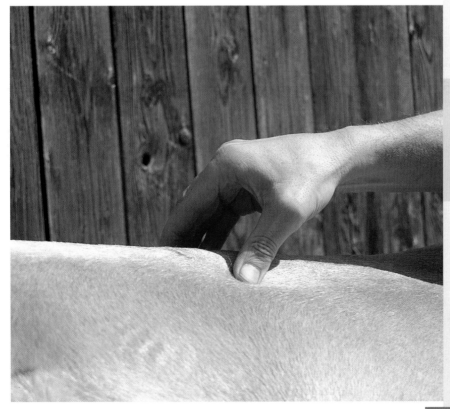

Direct pressure from the thumbs is suitable for treating small areas and is the chosen technique for trigger-point therapy and acupressure.

Using the index and middle fingers is another way to apply pressure on the tissues.

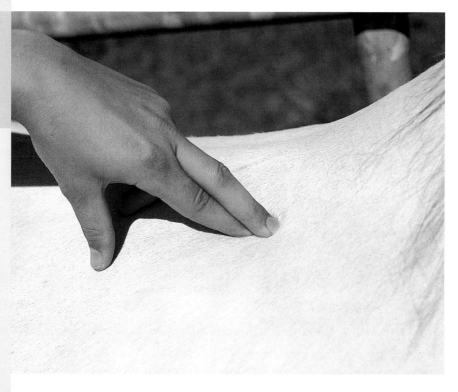

Using two hands to apply pressure.

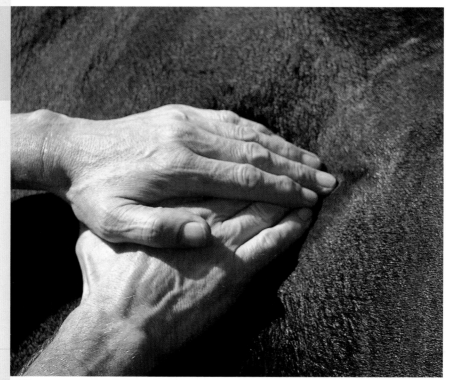

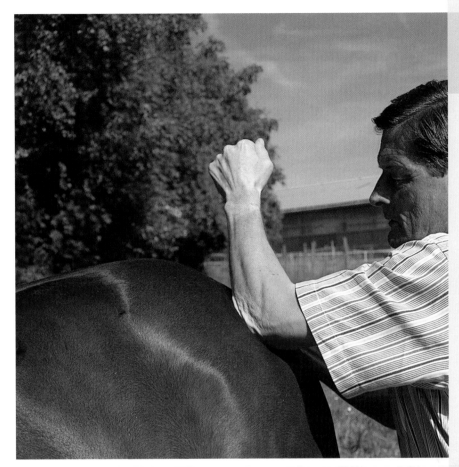

that the hand has more feeling for the pressure and effect on the horse. Once you know the technique and function of a movement, you can apply it with the brush as well.

Direct pressure

Direct pressure can be administered using various techniques. Thumbs are frequently used in this technique for strength and precision and the possibility of working in small areas. One or two fingers can also be used, sometimes even with support from the other hand.

When working on big groups of muscles and deeper layers, the elbow can be usefully applied for direct pressure.

The pressure is then sustained by putting one's body weight behind the elbow. The elbow technique is mainly used in the hindquarters, where the pressure is slowly increased and applied for 20-60 seconds. The intention is to relax the muscle and promote the flow of blood and furthermore to assess the amount of tension in the relevant muscles.

Direct pressure is also applied in trigger-point therapy where cross-friction and shifting is additionally put into service. Acupressure treatment employs finger pressure to stimulate acupressure points.

In classical massage, direct pressure is used to loosen tissues and knots caused by tension. The amount of pressure used depends on the muscle and the state of tension although you should aim mainly to apply less pressure.

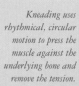

Kneading uses rhythmical, circular motion to press the muscle against the underlying bone and remove the tension.

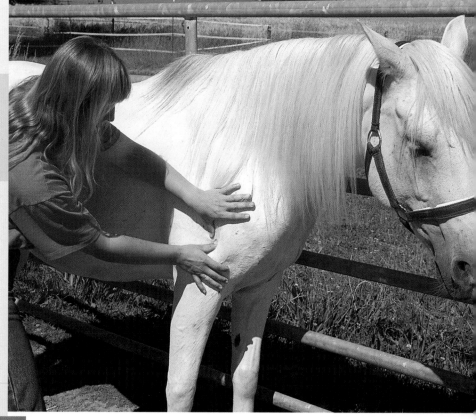

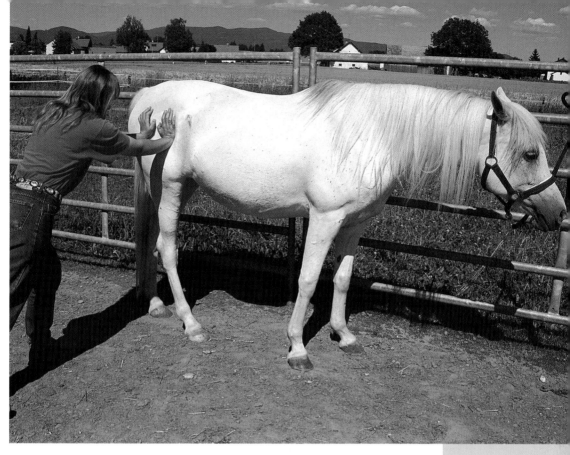

Direct pressure varies from compression and kneading, in that there is no rhythm or gliding across the muscles.

The pressure on the muscles has a calming effect on the horse if done slowly. Energetic pressure on the muscles has an energising effect, stimulating blood flow and warming the muscles, which means it can be a supplement to the warm-up phase of training.

Used as the relaxation massage, direct pressure can be excellent on the crest of the neck. Most horses enjoy this and will lower their heads to it. With extremely tense and sensitive muscles, however, great care must be taken and very little pressure used.

Rolling and kneading

There are numerous techniques for rolling and kneading. These techniques are dependent on the muscle that is worked on. You take the muscle between thumbs and

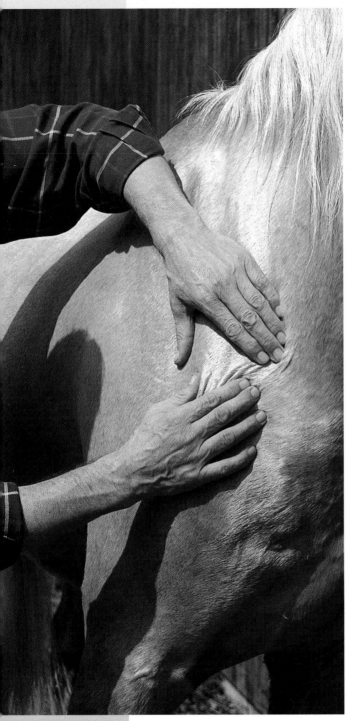

Wringing involves moving the hands in opposite directions.

fingers and push the tissue with the thumbs, supported by the balls of the hands. This technique is prescribed especially for the brachiocephalicus and hamstrings. In areas where the muscles are flatter, for example in the shoulder area, the hand is held flatter to knead with thumbs only. Using your own body weight in this technique increases the pressure on the muscles.

In using rolling and kneading the muscle is pushed against the bone underneath and compressed, proceeding in rhythmical, circular moves. The slower the movements are made, the more relaxing the massage. Faster rhythms and aggressive kneading increase the heart rate and rouse the horse.

Pettrisage (kneading) is, like the stroking movement, one of the basic movements that is used frequently. It is a movement to loosen tension, knots and spasms and to locate these muscular changes.

Kneading mobilises the muscles, returns them to their optimal tautness and transports excess liquid out of the tissue. Lumps can also be removed successfully with the use of kneading.

The strength of the pressure is between 1kg and 10 kg. As always, you start with light pressure and increase it steadily, depending on the amount demanded by the horse. Big, heavy horses can stand more pressure than small, lean horses. When horses are too fat, the physical force has to be

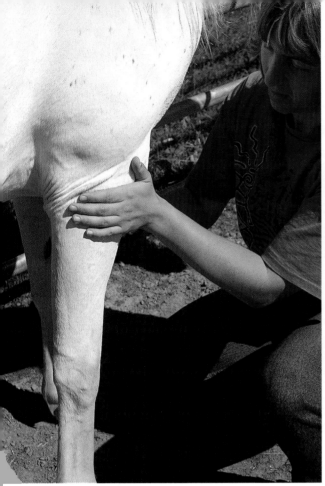
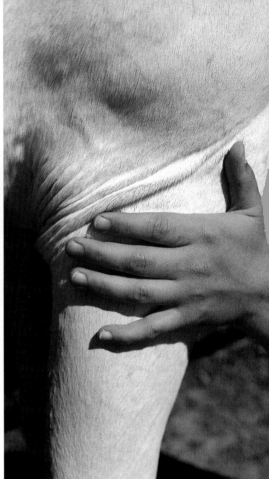

Lift the muscle in the direction of the fibres and press them against the bone.

much greater to be transferred through the extra layers. A massage does not therefore have the same effect on horses that are too fat.

Compression

Compression is a continuation of kneading, differing in that the muscles are not pushed over the underlying bone, but merely pressed against it. Compression can be executed with the fists or the ball of the hand. Input from your body weight can increase the pressure up to 15kg, helping to remove waste products by circulating fresh blood to the deeper-lying tissues. Compression is only used on big groups of muscle.

The aim of compression is relaxation, relieving spasms, preventing adhesions and knots and mobilisation of the muscles.

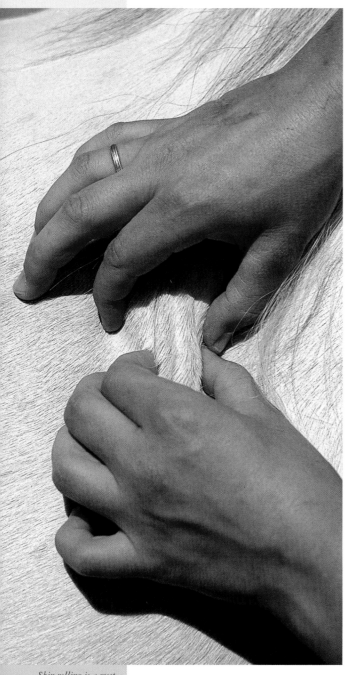

The same rule applies for compression as to all the others: working fast and aggressive-will stimulate the horse; long, slow strokes will relax the horse.

Wringing

This is an excellent movement for warming up the muscles. You use both hands, lay them flat on the body of the horse and move them in opposite directions. This can be used on the whole body. Protruding muscles are really suitable for wringing, as you can get a better hold of them. However, proceeding in a sensitive way will give you the best results.

Wringing is an excellent way to increase the blood flow, stimulating the removal of waste products and preventing tension. Muscles that profit most from wringing are the back, shoulders and hindquarters. It is important to find the correct rhythm that suits the horse and the situation.

Wringing is a marvellous way to end a loosening massage or to commence a cooling-down massage after training. They can be incorporated in the relaxation and maintenance massage where the slow rhythm is preferred.

Skin rolling is a most agreeable technique, where a crease is formed between the thumbs and fingers and pushed forward.

Lifting

In lifting, the muscle is pushed along the direction of fibre and compressed. You grasp the muscle with both hands, apply pressure and push the muscle as far as possible in the direction of its origin.

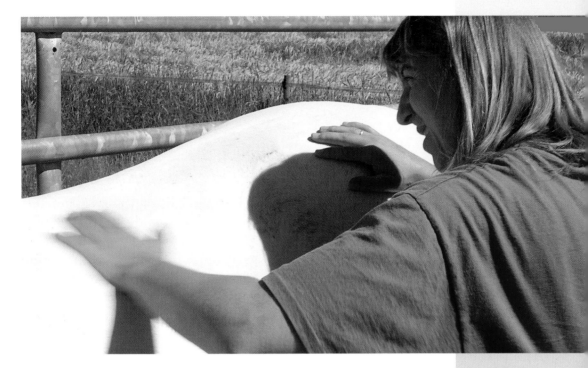

A fast vibration with the hand shifts the skin and stimulates the horse.

The pressure is maintained for a while and slowly released to glide back in its original position. This is to be repeated five to ten times.

Shake and wake

Vibrations and shaking increase muscle tone, waking the horse and preparing it for training or competing.

The muscles that are most suitable for lifting are those of the legs and the upper neck. Improved circulation is achieved and the muscles are brought into optimum basic tone. This technique is suitable for the loosening massage as it mobilises the muscles and prepares them for the training that lies ahead.

Skin rolls

This technique requires some practice. Using both hands, you push the skin between the fingers to make a crease. The fingers then pull and slightly lift the skin while the

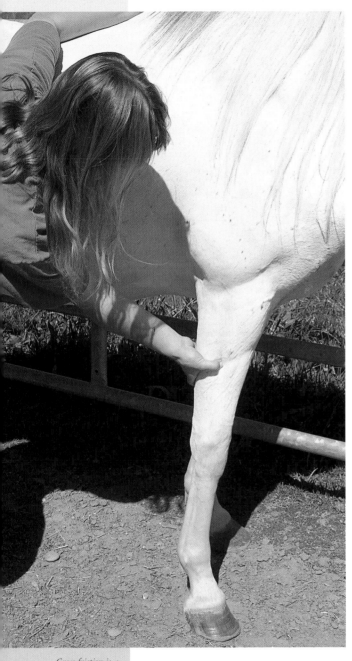

Cross friction is a sports therapy technique used to release adhesions. It is mainly done with the thumbs rubbing diagonally across the muscle fibres.

thumb presses lightly against it. The thumbs will then push the crease forward.

Another technique is to put both hands flat next to each other and push a crease between them. This crease can be pushed any direction you like, which makes it just as effective.

Rolling the skin is a gentle technique that is very agreeable and can be used anywhere on the body and in any direction. Skin rolling increases the circulation and elasticity of the skin, keeping the skin healthy, and can be employed to loosen adhesions (e.g. scar tissue after injury).

Shaking and vibration

Shaking and vibration is performed with one hand only. There are two different ways of doing this, the first utilising a flat hand. The hand is flat on the body with light pressure and moved fast from left to right. The contact with the body stays and the hand is not moved over the skin, but the skin is displaced over the underlying structures. The pressure used is approximately 1kg. The faster the vibration, the more stimulating the effect.

The second variation is to apply vibration using the fingertips.

The amount of pressure used is in the area of 2kg and is frequently used on localised muscular contractions to help them to relax.

Vibration massage on fingertips also stimulates the acupressure points that are in the deeper layers.

This massage is very calming on the nervous system when performed slower.

Deeper-lying muscles can be reached with vibrations and shaking. This technique stimulates and wakes the horse, increases blood flow, thus making it the perfect massage before training or competing.

Vibration on the legs can have very positive effects on the joints, especially where there are signs of arthritic changes or rheumatic conditions. Vibration is also excellent in the prevention of adhesions.

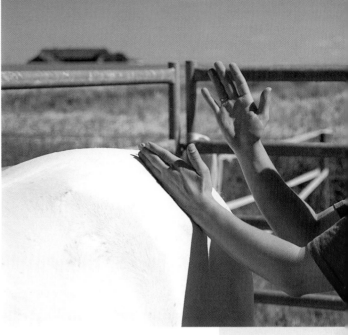

Hacking is extremely stimulating and done with the side of the hands.

Cupping is another technique of percussion.

Cross-friction

This technique involves diagonally shifting the skin over the underlying muscle fibres. Friction is also applied to tendons and ligaments, using the thumbs and fingertips.

This massage works very deeply and the pressure used is relatively high (5-10kg). Great care should be taken when applying this technique.

You should not interfere with any nerves or blood vessels, but only work on the tendons, ligaments and muscles.

The skin is pushed back and forth with strong pressure from the fingers and repeated 20 times before returning to a softer rubbing technique. After approximately 30 seconds this is repeated with even more pressure. This procedure should only be done for a few minutes in order not to irritate the tissue.

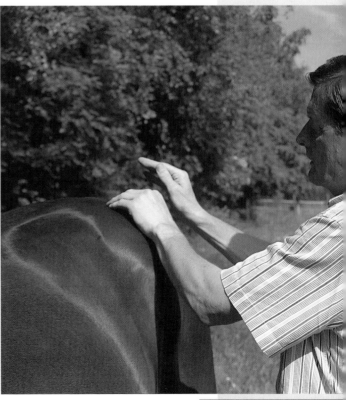

Cross-friction is a sport therapy technique that releases adhesions and should not be used until the area is sufficiently warmed up. This can be done with wringing, shaking, kneading or stroking. If cross-friction is exaggerated it can cause inflammation that can be painful for the horse. Friction should be done for no more than five minutes.

Cross-friction has an extremely therapeutic effect on blood flow, reduces pain and releases muscles and adhesions. It has a therapeutic purpose and must be performed in conjunction with ample stroking movements.

Percussion

This is a technique where both hands are used alternately to softly "chop" the body of the horse. You can use either a flat hand with palms facing (hacking), or a slightly rounded hand (cupping) and rhythmically chop the body, using pressure of 2-5 kg.

If the horse seems concerned about this technique (many horses have to learn to accept this), you can lessen the pressure and chop slower.

Percussion is only used on the bigger muscle groups; bony areas must be avoided. Percussion also includes beating with a soft fist, increasing the effect, but thus is seldom used.

These techniques are immensely stimulating and are therefore suitable to prepare the horse for training.

These movements are mainly used in the sports massage for they increase the circulation and intensify the muscle tone. Percussion can be used in the loosening massage for it contributes to the warming up.

The fist should only be used when you have already warmed the body with cupping and hacking. Beating with the fist works very deep, can irritate the horse and cause tension to become even stronger and should be used by a more experienced masseur only.

Basic principles of massage

You will have realised by now that massage is not meant as a bit of fun with your horse but that it is a treatment that has a specific effect. The horse can react to the treatment in a negative or positive way.

Practice makes perfect

To become a good masseur you need a great deal of practice

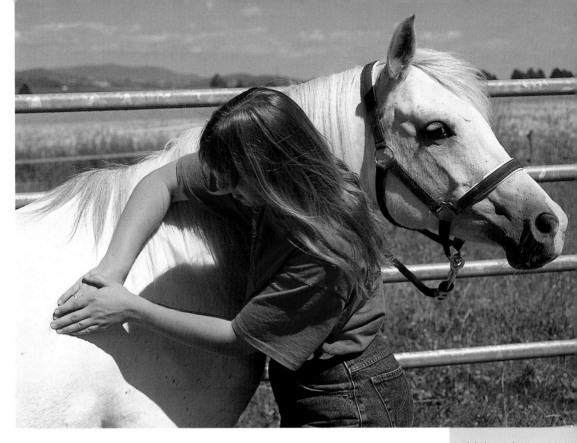

Most massage techniques have positive results, but they have to be purposefully employed. It is, for example, not advisable to give a horse a relaxing massage where the horse becomes drowsy just before a demanding cross-country competition. In this case the performance capability will be lowered instead of increased. Increasing the performance would have been influenced had the horse been given a stimulating massage with percussion and vibrations.

It is therefore not prudent to merely stroke and knead around and hope that it will be good for the horse. You have to have an intimate knowledge of the muscles, tendons and bones of the horse and understand what the effects of the movements are. There are further criteria incorporated as well.

Pressure and speed

As mentioned earlier on, each horse is sensitive in its own way to feeling, pressure and outside influences. One horse will find 2kg pressure too much on a specific point, while another might perceive it as just right.

The massage must be changed to adapt to the individual horse; the recommended pressure only serves as a guideline. The actual pressure and speed of the movements will be determined by the tactile sense of the masseur. In order to do this, you must learn to "read" the horse's reaction and mood.

Horses do not always jump aside when a movement is unpleasant, some of them will react in a totally different way. They can become disgruntled, irritated or simply tighten their muscles. This reaction is exactly what you do not want! Practice and experience will improve your feeling for the amount of pressure and speed called for in the movements.

Duration

These are only guidelines as to the length of a massage. If a muscle is tense it can relax after 30 seconds or after three minutes. The length of the massage also depends on what you want to achieve with it. If you want to treat localised areas it can be over within five to ten minutes whereas a whole body massage will take longer.

The length of the massage can be influenced by additional factors. If it is the first treatment for the horse, the massage should be kept short, as the horse might become restless if it does not know what to expect.

Once the horse shows that it is happy with the massage, the time can be extended. Once the horse is used to being massaged, a treatment can continue for an hour or more.

The massage after training or competition should take between 15 and 30 minutes, for the muscles can cool off and return to normal within this time.

When working on a localised area, for therapeutic purposes, the massage should not be longer than ten minutes, whether the goal was reached or not. Taking too long can irritate the tissue and make the problem worse, or even cause inflammation.

It is naturally also a question of whether you can or want to spend an hour massaging your horse.

Obviously you can keep the relaxation and the maintenance massage short, but do not expect 100% results from that. Sometimes it is better to concentrate on a specific area and treat that thoroughly, rather than massage the whole horse superficially.

It is always best to treat with a goal in mind, rather than massage in general. For this reason it is recommended to plan ahead and decide what technique to employ to reach what effect.

Safety

Although you have the horse's best interest at heart, the horse might react in a negative way once the massage is underway.

Kicking, biting and stamping the feet are some of the ways a horse shows discomfort. Not every horse enjoys a massage and you have to be prepared for any eventuality. Adhesions and spasms are painful and when you try to treat them the horse might react, from pure reflex, in a dangerous way.

You must therefore always be on your guard when massaging a horse. This applies right at the beginning, when assessing the horse, and in the way you approach the horse. Contact should be taken up first on the neck, and from here you work yourself to the area that you want to work on, keeping a steady contact on the body with the hands.

Your working technique must be appropriate to minimise the safety risk. Make sure the space you work in is big enough, that there are no wheelbarrows, hayforks, buckets or other objects that you or the horse may trip over or get injured by.

Make sure the surroundings are quiet and peaceful: continuous bustle is not the desired atmosphere to relax in.

Children playing, dogs running and a radio playing loud music can all be disturbing to both the horse and the masseur.

The horse can react in an unpredictable way even if the surroundings are ideal, so you must always concentrate on your work and the possible reactions of the horse. The posture of the masseur must be stable, feet slightly apart and knees bent, always keeping contact with the horse via the hands. If one hand is not used in the treat-

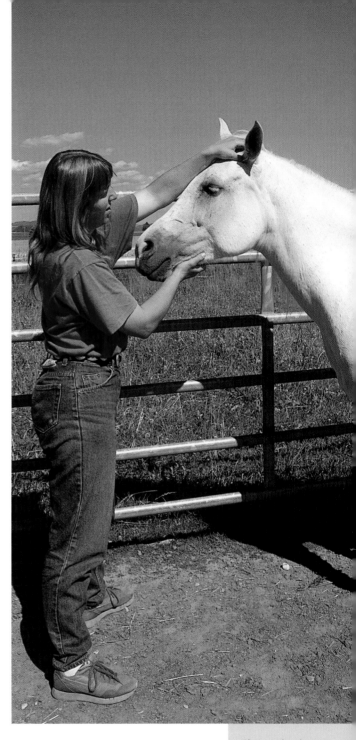

Choose a calm, pleasant spot where you can work in peace.

ment, rest it on the body of the horse, this way you will feel when the horse is going to react and can get out of the way safely.

It is recommended to wear comfortable clothing that is neither too tight nor too loose. More important is that you must wear shoes that will protect your feet from those hooves!

Contra-indications

There are some cases where a massage has a negative effect on the horse. The best advice is to leave it be when you are not sure whether a massage will do good or not. The vet must always be consulted when injury or illness is present.

If the horse has a fever, it should not be massaged. The normal temperature of the horse is 37.5–38.2 degrees Celsius. If the horse has a fever, the blood flow is already higher, which means that a massage will only make the situation worse.

A further contra-indication is an acute injury or open wound.

You can bypass these areas and massage the rest of the body. Under no circumstances should you massage an injured area that is warm and swollen, for this is painful for the horse and will make the injury worse. Sprains and strains are also injuries that are contra-indicated.

Do not massage when a horse has a skin infection, e.g. eczema, fungal or parasite infestation. The same applies for tumours, cancerous lumps or cysts.

Horses with infectious diseases should be left alone, purely due to the danger of infecting other horses, for this is often accompanied by fever and this is already good reason not to massage a horse.

Massage in practice

You should have a general picture of the horse before you start to massage it. Is it ill? Is it calm or excited? Does it have an injury or another problem?

Then you decide what type of massage would be appropriate. Should the excited horse have a relaxing massage? Do you need to do a loosening massage just before training? Maybe there is no specific reason for a massage, in which case the maintenance massage will be all right.

When you know of specific problems, you can do a partial massage on that particular area.

Applied technique

The massage is determined by the pressure applied, rhythm and speed and then of course by the way the masseur uses the techniques.

The feeling of the masseur will decide what technique to use, how fast, how long and with what intensity, all of which will be increased with practice.

The area of the body normally determines the techniques used, but the type of techniques does not always determine the result of the massage. It is more the pressure used, rhythm and speed that determine the outcome. It is important to know what you want to achieve; concentrating while you treat will bring the best results.

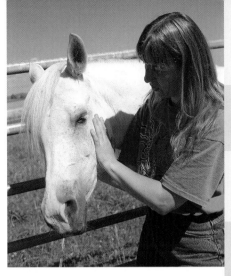

You start the head massage with soft stroking on the cheeks.

You continue with stroking on the bridge of the nose.

Head and neck

Suspicious horses will not enjoy having their faces being massaged right away, especially not by some stranger. If you have a good relationship with your horse and it is used to having its head touched, however it will probably have no problem having its face thoroughly massaged.

When massaging the face you must be extra careful for there are numerous nerves, blood vessels, reflex points and bones directly beneath the skin.

It is precisely because of these sensitive areas on the face that you can achieve a wonderfully relaxing massage that influences the whole body. You start the massage with slow stroking on the cheeks and the bridge of the nose.

The massage continues with pressing the muscles at the base of the ear and the poll, using one hand on this side, the other on the other side.

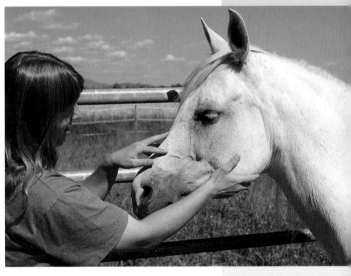

Massage of the poll and base of the ears has an extremely relaxing effect.

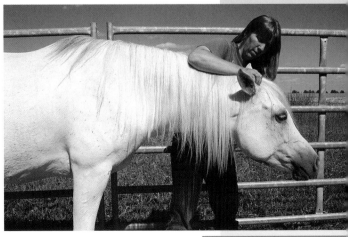

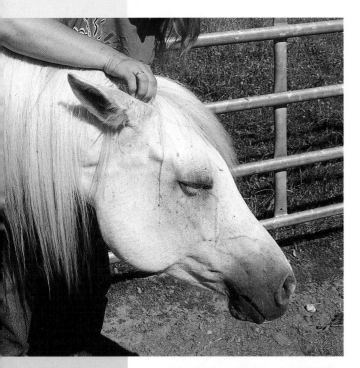

This Arab mare obviously enjoys the massage on the poll.

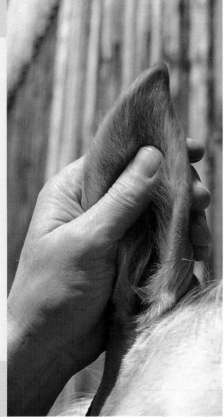

Softly stroking the inside of the ear increases relaxation.

Proceed to the forehead, stroking between the eyes with circular movements. The medial corner of the eye has neurovascular points that can be stimulated to relax and which act as drainage for the eye.

Next you move on to the mouth area, where massaging the top lip and gums has a calming influence on the horse through the release of endorphins. If horses do not enjoy being touched around the mouth, do not insist on doing so.

The cheek muscles of the horse do a tremendous amount of work when the horse chews and problems with the teeth make the situation worse. If the problem of a rider with a hard hand is added to that, you can guarantee tension in the masseter muscle.

Using hand stroking and very soft kneading will loosen some of the tension. From here you return to the ear and poll area. When the horse accepts the touch at the ears you can softly stroke the inside of the ears and repeat this for up to ten times.

The head massage should be for no longer than ten minutes and from there you move to the neck with long strokes. These long effleurage strokes will lead to the horse lowering its neck.

This will unclench the muscles. Now you can knead the crest of the mane and execute small circles along the vertebrae of the neck. Pull the big muscle on the bottom of the neck towards yourself while pushing the crest of the mane away from you to include the whole neck and to conclude the massage on the neck.

Chest, shoulders and forehand

A flowing continuation of stroking will bring you to the chest and shoulder. Preventive massage with kneading, compression and shaking can be employed on the chest, and stroking down in the direction of the heart can drain the excess liquid. This should take in the region of five minutes.

The shoulder is attached to the horse with muscles and ligaments. This means that the range of movement is totally dependent on the suppleness of the shoulder. Once the muscles of the shoulder are

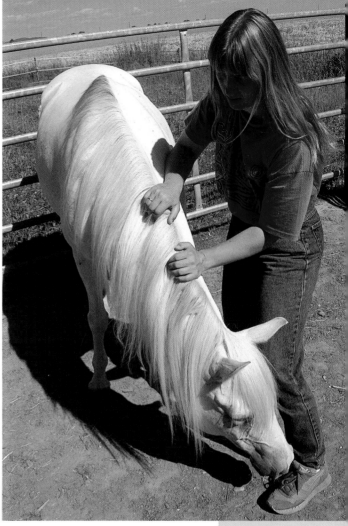

Once the horse is relaxed you can knead the crest of the neck.

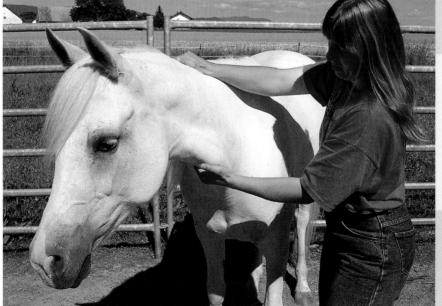

For even more relaxation you can pull the brachiocephalicus muscle towards yourself while at the same time pushing the crest of the neck away.

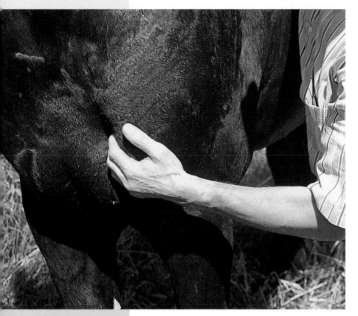

You can treat the chest area with kneading and pressing of the muscles.

The grip behind the shoulder shows whether the shoulder muscles are relaxed.

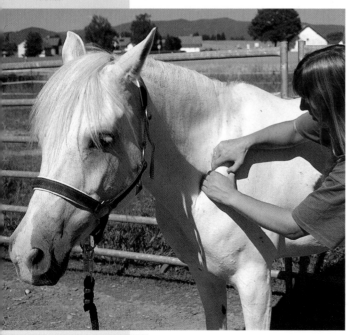

tensed up (mainly the ones that attach behind the shoulder), the horse's athleticism is decreased. In extreme cases lameness can be the result.

The massage on the shoulders is started with soft thumb-kneading alternated with slow, long effleurage strokes.

When the horse is being massaged before training or competing, you can apply extensive shaking; after exercise, soft kneading and wringing has a better effect.

Once the muscles are warmed up, you stroke up and down the shoulder and try to tuck your hand behind the shoulder blade. If the muscles are relaxed, it is possible to tuck the whole hand behind the shoulder blade. This is made easier by encouraging the horse to bend its head slightly to the side you are working on.

Stroking then takes you on to the front legs. The "C-grip" and lifting is suitable to warm and loosen tension on the lower leg. Using wringing and kneading you slowly work your way down the leg. There are no muscles below the carpal joint, only tendons, ligaments and bone, and these calls for special care. Upward stroking helps drain liquid out of the leg below the fetlock.

The draining technique is mainly applied on the inside of the leg.

Treatment of the back and barrel
Moving from the back up to the withers is where you start the back massage. The maintenance massage

incorporates kneading, interspersed with effleurage to promote relaxation. This area is extremely prone to tension, not only from poorly fitting saddles, but also through "leakage" from the shoulder area.

Hand stroking bridges the distance to the back muscles, where you can start thumb kneading or wringing. This can be extended to the barrel and helps to drain the ribs. Pay attention always to drain in the direction of the heart.

Shaking in the back and rib areas will wake the horse and promote blood flow to these areas. Percussion can then follow and this can be used to perk up a tired horse and increase the muscle tone. All these movements are followed by effleurage.

If relaxation is your goal, the withers are treated with soft kneading, while on the back only soft stroking or wringing is applied. These strokes are done to cover a large area over the whole barrel.

Tension between the ribs can be loosened with direct pressure, kneading and vibrations.

Skin rolling can be put into service on large areas to promote flow of blood and relaxation. This is once more concluded with effleurage.

Hindquarters

The hands glide over the croup to the hindquarters. Movements that can be employed on these extensive muscles include kneading, direct pressure, and compressions, including the elbow technique for more effectiveness.

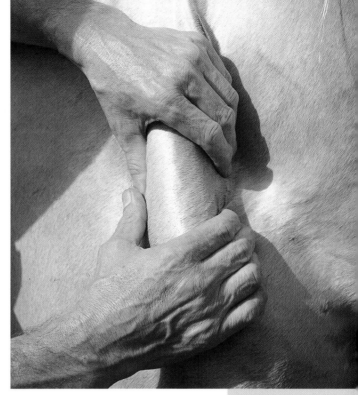

Softly lifting the shoulder blade helps loosen tense muscles in the shoulder area.

Stroking on the inside of the lower leg in an upward direction drains the liquid.

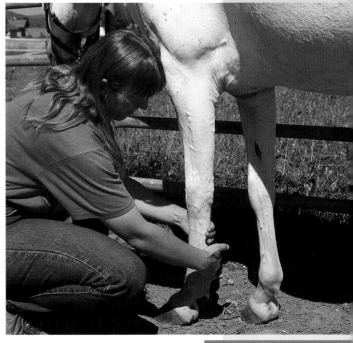

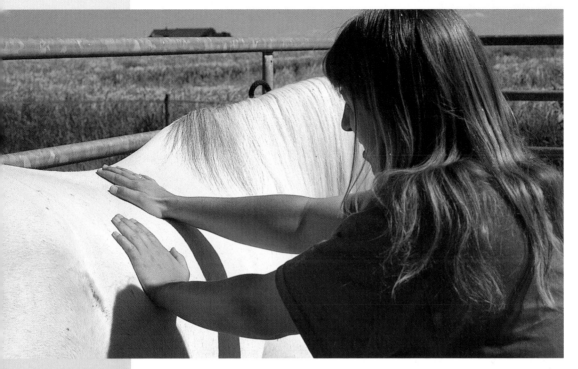

To prepare the horse for exercise you can use the wringing technique.

Big stroking movements on the barrel relax the horse.

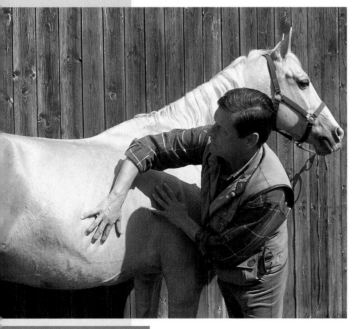

Using both hands you can then massage around the bony areas of the seat bones but be careful, this area can be tender and the horse may react with a mighty kick! From the seat bone down you can use the C-grip on the knee, paying attention to the sensitivity of the horse.

The hamstrings (semitendinosus and semimembranosus) are treated with pressure to relieve tension and spasms. These muscles are often tight in Western horses and jumpers. For competition these muscles are treated with compression, wringing and shaking to achieve an optimum state of tautness. The

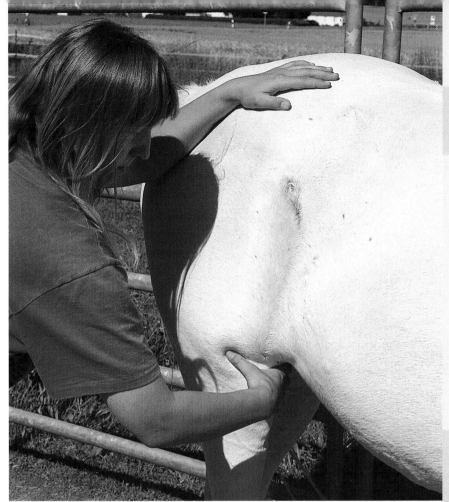

The long muscles at
the hind end are
treated with pressure
to release tension and
spasms.

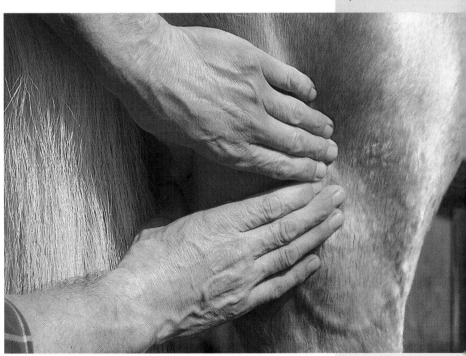

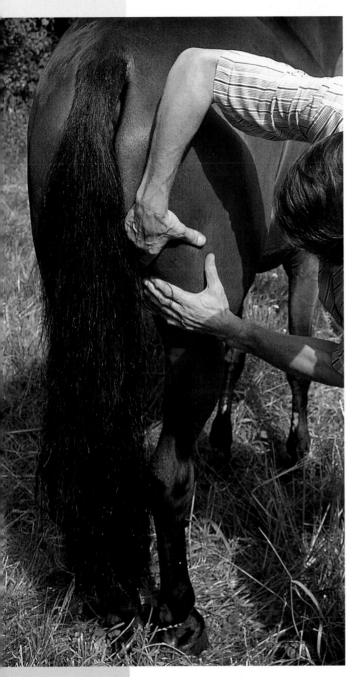

Western horses and jumpers often have tight muscles at the hind end and require special attention.

lower leg lends itself to lifting, wringing, kneading and compression.

Below the hock you will use the stroking technique in an upward direction, just as on the front legs.

Techniques for the tail

Manipulating the tail can be used to advantage in the relaxing massage. Manoeuvring the tail can be extremely positive for the muscles of the back and hindquarters.

Take the tail in your hand, just below the dock (for your safety, it is better not to stand directly behind the horse) and lift the tail up. If the horse is relaxed, this is very easy to do. Do not force this action but rather return to more relaxing massage before attempting to do this again.

If it is easy to lift the tail, rotate it to one side and then to the other. You can also make a circle, once in each direction.

If you notice any restriction in the movement, this may point to tension in the back or hindquarters. When too little movement is present, take the tail from behind and pull it slowly to stretch the muscles between the vertebrae. Under normal circumstances the horse will lean away in the opposite direction, resulting in a super stretch for the topline.

You can put your whole body weight behind the pull, providing you start slowly and release it slowly. It is often necessary for two or three people to put a proper

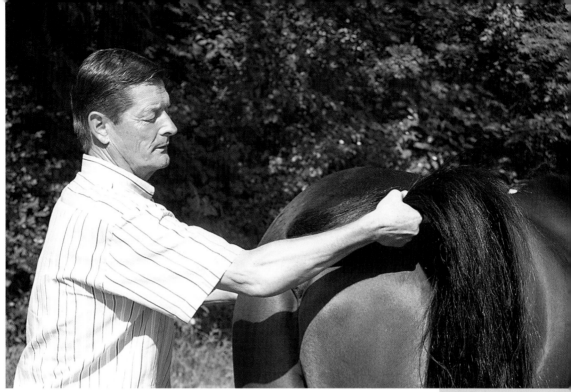

stretch on the tail, keeping the stretch for 20-30 seconds and slowly releasing it. Many horses enjoy this and will lower their heads to the ground. The single vertebrae of the tail can be pressed, and lifting and rotating of the tail can be done once more after the pull.

Conclude the massage with slow effleurage over the whole body of the horse.

The tail is carefully lifted and rotated to assess the mobility.

Slowly increase the weight behind the pull of the tail, using the whole body weight to reach a proper stretch.

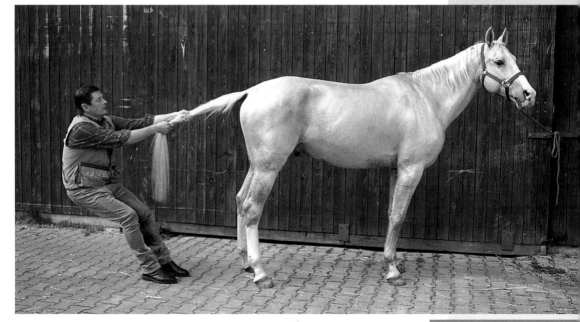

VI

Stretches

Effects and goals of stretches

Stretches are the perfect completion of a massage aiding in the relaxation produced by the massage. They stimulate blood flow, increase mobility and elasticity of the muscles, tendons and ligaments, and improve coordination and flexibility of the joints. The potential for injury is also reduced with stretching.

For the best results, stretching should be done after a massage or after training, when the muscles are warm. You risk injuries like pulling or tearing the muscles when they are stretched cold. When stretching follows the warm-up massage, the horse will be well prepared for training or competition. Stretching

after training will have a positive effect on the training of the next day.

Stretching is part of any athletic activity and is done immediately after warming up. This tried and tested way should become an element of your horse's training as well.

Stretching will improve the performance of the horse, for it minimises the risk of injury and prepares the muscles to fulfil their task.

Muscles are dependent on their opposing partners: when an agonist tightens, it can only tighten as far as the antagonist stretches out. Performance is therefore not only dependent on the strength of a muscle but also the flexibility.

Passive and active stretching

There are two ways of stretching active and passive. With active stretching the agonist muscle tightens in order for its antagonist to stretch.

Passive stretching involves the strength of outside influences while the agonist stays relaxed. This outside influence in the case of the horse

---

Performance of muscles

Flexible muscles function better with their opposing partners, stretching further when the opposing muscle tightens. Flexibility and strength are two important components for the ability of muscles to perform.

---

is the human being. In many cases groups of muscles can be stretched from "outside" using other muscles: for example, pulling up the toes will stretch the muscles of the calves. Unfortunately you cannot teach the horse to do this by itself.

The horse is often not convinced that it should do some of the active stretches for it cannot understand the reason behind it. This is where treats can help with the exercise.

Passive stretching is much more effective than active stretching, for the wilful tightening of the agonist does not always mean the antagonist will stretch to its maximum capacity. Passive stretching has a more relaxing effect on the muscle for there is no opposing stretch.

You should be aware that passive stretching can be dangerous when not executed with care. Every

muscle has so called receptors that register and supervise the length of the muscle. If there is any danger of overstretching, these receptors will react with a fast reflex that contracts the muscle in order for it not to hurt itself.

This protecting reflex is only available in a restricted form when passive stretching is performed. Passive stretching is on the one hand a fantastic way to lengthen the muscles, but on the other hand must be practised with care as potentially it can be quite dangerous as well.

Once you have ample experience in massage you can try your hand at passive stretching; if not, it is safer to start with the active stretching exercises where the treats are used.

Techniques for stretching

A stretch is only effective when it is held for a minimum of ten seconds. This is not always possible with active stretching: either the horse has already eaten the treat or it loses interest when you keep the treat just out of its reach for a long time. This is only one reason why active stretching is not as effective.

With passive stretching you extend a limb, for example, until you reach a resistance. This position is then held until the resistance slackens. This will take approximately 10-30 seconds. Then you take up the slack and stretch the muscle a little further until you reach some resistance once more. Now you stretch the muscle for another 10-30 seconds. Relax the stretch comple te-

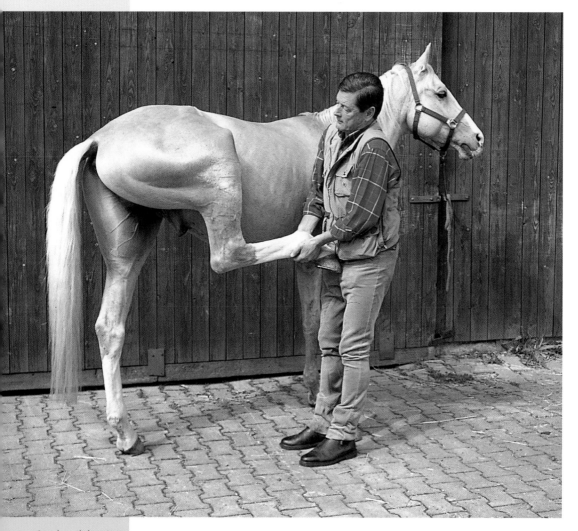

Stretch until the resist-ance goes; this takes approximately 10-30 seconds.

ly and then repeat it three or four times.

Stretching must not be done in haste, for this can lead to overstretch-ing. Do not bounce the limb, for the maximum stretch cannot be reached this way and the bounce has a con-traction reflex that makes the whole exercise pointless.

If the horse becomes fidgety or pulls the limb away, the stretching

capacity is lessened. This could be because the horse does not trust the masseur, or because there is tension and spasms that are pain-ful. With nervous horses extra time has to be taken to massage them (sometimes more than once) until you have achieved the state of relaxation that produces trust in the masseur.

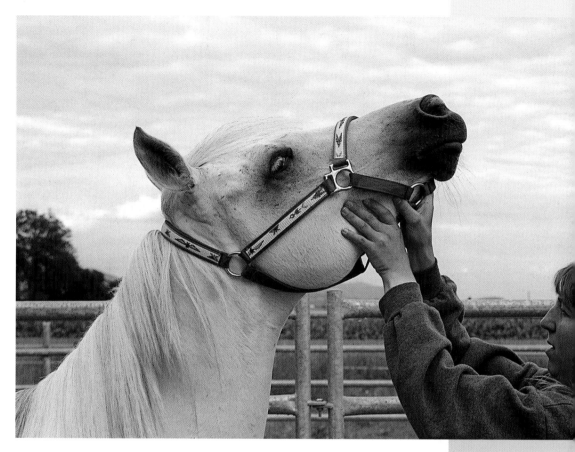

Stretching in practice

Naturally you are only allowed to do stretches on healthy horses, for it can worsen some injuries.

Stretching is contra-indicated when there is fever, inflammation, open wounds and all the reasons where a massage is also not allowed.

Horses have massive bodies with relatively heavy limbs, so a certain amount of power is asked for. You should always be careful to protect your own body, for example by keeping your back straight and using your leg muscles to take up some of the weight. You must always be aware that the horse can struggle against the stretch and might react in a dangerous way.

Accidents can be avoided with correct footwear, good clothes (not too loose or too tight) and if you work in a safe and quiet area.

The neck stretch

Good flexibility of the neck muscles increases the horse's athletic ability, balance and agility. Stiffness or lack of flexibility influences the condition of the rest of the body.

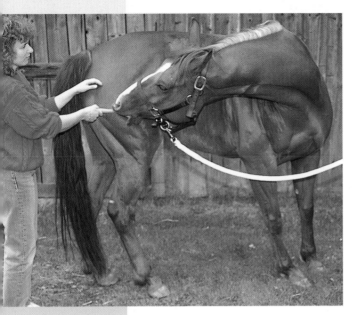

Stretching to the side is achieved in an active way by offering a treat in the region of the croup.

poll. If the horse bends its nose down to the vertical, the goal is achieved. Many horses will move back with pressure on the nose so it is a good idea to put the backside of the horse against a wall to counter-act this.

To stretch all the muscles at the top of the neck the horse's nose must be lowered to its chest. This is an active stretch that can be per-formed with the help of treats.

The opposing stretch to this is extending the horse's head in the opposite direction.

This can be done in an active or passive way. You can either hold a treat in front of the nose (active) or push the head up with the hands under the chin (passive).

Extending the neck to the side can be done actively or passively, once again, leading the head with a treat or putting a hand on the nose to push the neck to the shoulder.

If you want to include the shoulder and rump muscles you can extend the head towards the hipbone. To prevent the horse from stepping to the side you can put it next to a wall.

To stretch the neck of the horse, you put your hands on the bridge of the horse's nose and with light pressure the horse should bend its

Extending the neck to the side can also be achieved with passive stretching.

Exercises for the limb

Effective work on the limbs can only be achieved when the horse can balance on three legs. If this is not the case the horse will tense up its muscles or fight the stretch.

It is also easier to start with the front legs. Pick up the hoof as if you want to pick it, then take the upper arm and move the leg to the front until the full capacity of the stretch is reached.

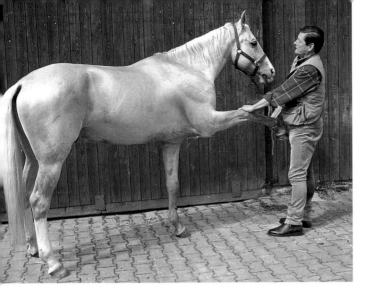

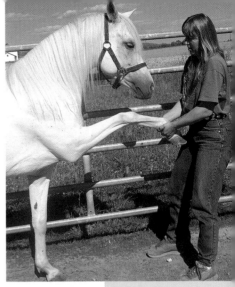

Left: In stretching the front leg you will involve the wide back muscle, the flexors and deltoid muscle.

Right: The leg is held at the fetlock.

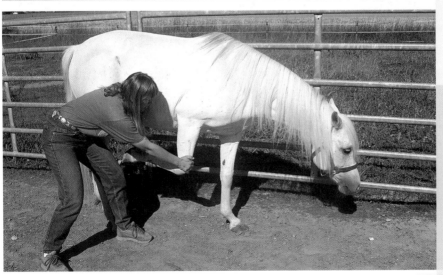

To protect the carpal joint you can hold the leg at the forearm and let the cannon bone hang down.

To stretch the brachiocephalicus, extensors and chest muscles, the leg is pulled back. Putting a hand on the forearm protects the carpal joint.

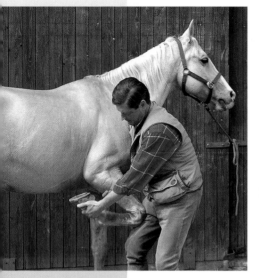

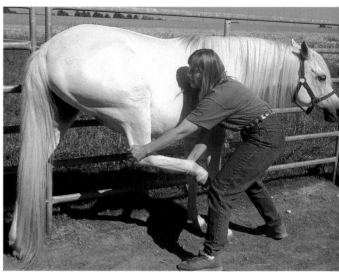

Left: To protect your own body, you can put the knee of the horse on your thigh and push the leg back.

Right: The hand supports the back leg on the stifle joint.

In this way you achieve a stretch of the big back muscle, triceps, deltoids as well as the flexors.

The leg is held at the fetlock. The alternative is to hold the leg at the forearm and let the cannon hang down, but this stretch is slightly less as the ligaments continue right down to the hoof.

To lengthen the extensors, the brachiocephalicus and chest muscles you have to draw the front leg backwards.

You take the carpal joint in one hand, the fetlock joint in the other and pull the leg back. Pressure comes only from the hand on the carpal joint. An easy variation for

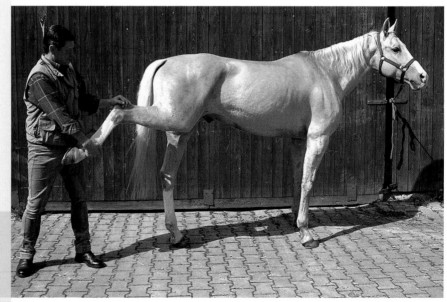

The quadriceps, extensors and adductors are stretched when the leg is extended backwards.

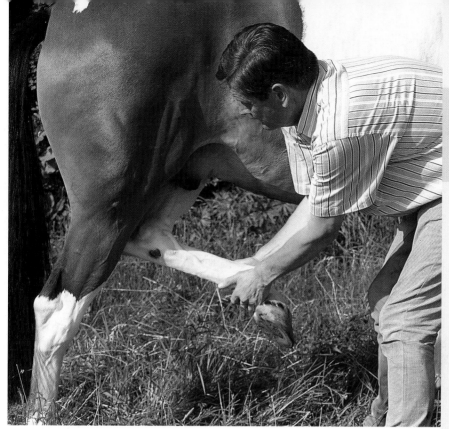

the therapist is to place the horse's knee on your thigh and extend the knee back with the weight of your own body.

To stretch the trapezius and rhomboid muscles, you pick up the front leg and cross it over the other leg.

The hoof must stay as close to the ground as possible when doing this stretch. Crossing over to the back of the leg will stretch the big back muscle.

Stretching the back leg is done in much the same way. You pick up the leg at the fetlock and stretch it to the front, extending all the muscles of the croup and the biceps femoris. Take care not to pull the leg out to the side, as this will put unnecessary strain on the joints.

To extend the leg to the back, you take the cannon bone in your hand and slowly lean backwards with your weight. This will stretch the quadriceps, extensors and adductors.

Crossing the back leg in front of the other one will extend the muscles of the croup, the hamstrings and the biceps femoris.

The back

A marvellously active back is the foundation for dynamic gaits and an athletic horse. The mere fact that the rider's weight pushes the back down makes it most important to practise correct training, stretching and strengthening of the back muscles.

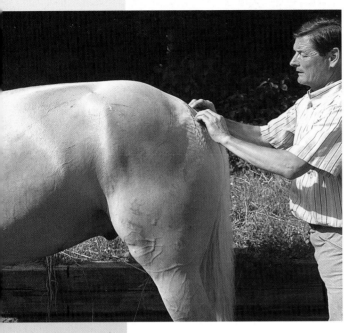

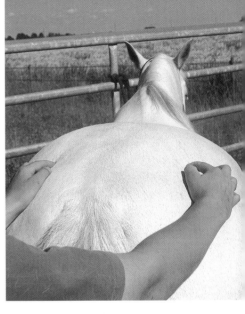

Left: Pressure on the reflex points on the croup will curve the back upwards.

Right: The reflex points in the croup area.

Seeing that the back muscles are the antagonists for the abdominal muscles, these two are directly linked with each other. Contraction of the abdominals will stretch the back muscles, and the other way round.

Stretching the foreleg already touches on these muscles. When you extend the foreleg to the back you will see how the back curves upwards and pulling the leg to the front you will incorporate some of the abdominals in the stretch, slightly hollowing the back.

Direct treatment of the back muscles can be achieved with the reflex points. Direct pressure on the breastbone will curve the back upwards, opening the spaces between the spinous processes of the vertebrae at the withers, thus stretching the back muscles. Pressure on the reflex points on the croup will curve the back in the loin area. These two reflex points will give you a complete stretch in the whole of the back.

When you only put pressure on one reflex point on the croup, the horse will stretch the side of the back. This stretch should always be combined with the pressure point at the breastbone. Sideways extension is a good stretch for the abdominal muscles.

Finding the reflex points

Stand behind the horse and slide your fingers over the croup muscles in the direction of the seat bone. This is the best way to find the reflex points that lift the loin vertebrae.

You will normally follow the direction of hair growth to trigger the reflex points for the back lift. An aggressive trigger can be achieved when going against the growth of the hair, but care must be taken not to overstretch the back. The ideal is when the back makes a straight line.

An excellent stretch for the back is to put the forelegs on an elevation (e.g. a platform)

A further outstanding stretch is when the horse stretches its head as far as possible between its legs. Use treats for this and make sure the horse only receives them once maximum stretch has been achieved. The difficulty of this exercise is that the horse must learn to spread its forelegs slightly for the head to pass through. Some practice is needed for this. Many clever horses will do this without treats, or on specific commands.

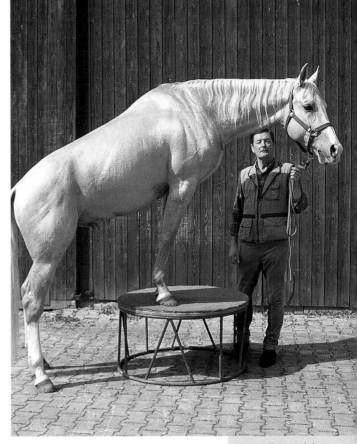

An excellent stretch for the back is to let the horse stand on a platform with the forelegs.

An active stretch for the back is to offer a treat between the front legs.

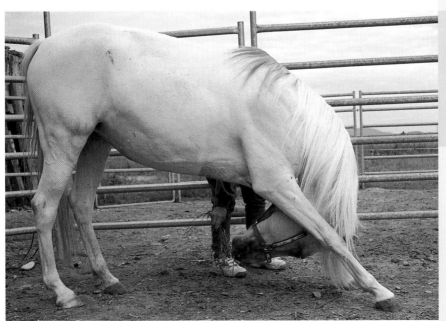

VII

Problem Areas

Demands on the horse

Almost everyone has some form of tension and adhesions, due to the unnatural way we live. This can be from bad posture at the work desk or even when out doing sports. The problem remains the same: repetitive movements that put too much strain on the body.

The situation with horses is not very different. We have even bred horses for very specific purposes. The cold-blooded horses were bred to pull heavy loads, thoroughbreds run like the wind and these warmbloods are employed in various disciplines of riding. Selection of breeds goes even deeper: for example, the Quarter horses for cutting, reining, and big warmbloods for dressage, and so on. Genetic selection may have lessened the over-taxation in certain areas of the body for particular purposes, but unfortunately cannot prevent it altogether. The specialisation of horses for disciplines will always be accompanied by health problems.

Sport horses
This is an area of definite specialisation, bringing with it specific injuries, illnesses and wear. This is where the breed does not play any role.

Jumpers are tremendously taxed in the hindquarters, not only from the muscular point of view, but also the tendons, ligaments and bones.

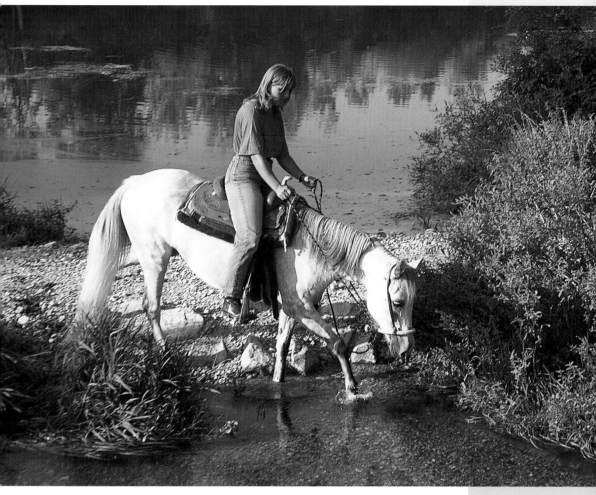

Variation in the routine of the horse can minimise tension and wear.

When the horse lands (on one leg!), having to take the whole weight is extremely arduous for the tendons, ligaments and bones. The chest and leg muscles are also rigorously punished in the process.

Dressage horses have problems in the hindquarters where they have to work in collection all the time. Strain is noticeable in the hock, knee, back and the muscles of the hindquarters.

Western horses have special problems, depending on the discipline. The hindquarters are severely taxed in reining, as are the back, shoulder and chest muscles.

Tension in the muscles is normally the first sign of a problem that can turn into a weakness if not treated rapidly.

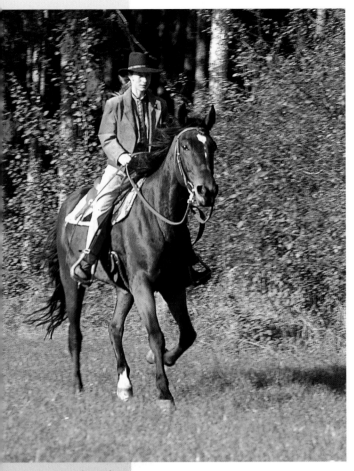

Leisure horses often suffer tension and wear if not trained properly and ridden by riders with insufficient skills.

The excessive demand made from riders with insufficient skill can lead to permanent damage of the horse. It is a shame that most of these riders do not even recognise the harm done. Many riders ask their horses to perform above their abilities and are not aware that the horses can suffer a lot of pain because of this.

Each rider has to learn how to ride and this is only possible on a horse. Having to cope with extreme demands – especially on the back (bouncing rider) and the neck (severe hands) – is almost inevitable for school horses.

The leisure horse, ridden regularly by an experienced, kind rider is lucky. Unfortunately this does not mean that the horse will be completely free of tension and wear. It is estimated that 90% of all problems are from the rider while 10% are from temperament, conformation, genetic and similar factors.

Leisure horses

The idea that leisure horses have an easier time is not always the case. Their owners often ride them at irregular intervals and every so often participate in a competition for which the horse is not properly prepared. It is also frequently the case that many of these riders are beginners.

Approach to treatment and therapy

When you include the breed, conformation, demands and (especially!) the ability of the rider in your assessment of the likelihood of problems, you have a greater chance of uncovering the possible problem areas. You can then devise a plan to solve or lessen some of the problems (a different saddle, or change of training). Lastly the problems can be minimised by specific massage and stretching exercises.

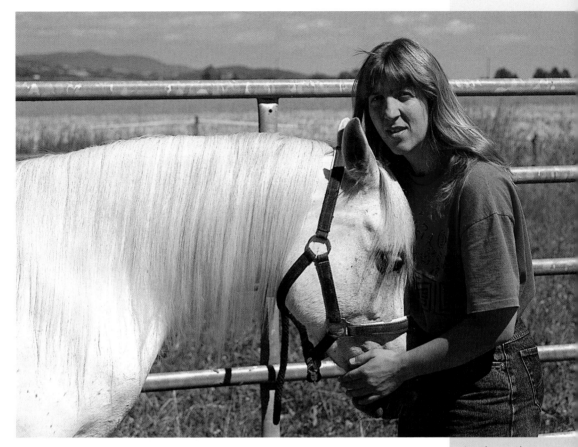

A good massage boosts the horse's well-being and stenghtens the relationship between man and animal.

No treatment, whether from a masseur or vet, can eliminate a problem if the reason for it is not removed. Treating a horse with massage, stretching exercises and other physiotherapy techniques can only support therapy and is not a solution to all problems. However, preventive massage can keep susceptible areas free from pain and improve freedom of movement.

The most important aspect of massage is that it promotes a feeling of well-being and strengthens the relationship between the horse and man on the physical and psychological levels.

Further reading

Bromiley -
(1996)Horse Massage,
Kenilworth Press

Denoix and Pailloux -
(1996) Physical Therapy and
Massage for Horses,
Manson Publishing

Gray, Peter -
(1993) Soundness in the Horse,
J.A. Allen

Hourdebaigt, Jean-Pierre -
(1997) Equine Massage,
Ringpress Books

Kamen, Dr Daniel -
(1999) The Well Adjusted Horse, Brookline Books, Cambridge
Mass.

Meagher, Jack -
-(1998) Beating Muscle Injuries
in Horses,
Cloudcrossed book

Olsen, Chris -
(2002) A Hot Line to Your Horse, Cadmos

Scott, Mike -
(1997) The Basic Principles of
Equine Massage, Muscle Therapy Productions, Bolton

Sutton, Amanda -
(2002) The Injury-free Horse,
David & Charles Ltd